Testimonials

"A perceptive and thorough analysis of our American diet, including insightful revelations about healthy eating, medical practices, and health education. This should be required reading for all school district decision makers. This message is too important to let it go unnoticed."

Jon Erlandson
A Founder of Healthy Food in Schools

"I love the comprehensive scope of this book and think every chapter and topic is important for readers to consider! Thank you for sticking up for plant-based protein! Thank you for sticking up for carbs!"

Laurie Powell
Doctor of Psychology
Plant-Based Nutritionist
Health Educator

"Honest information from an expert dietitian and health educator in the field for over thirteen years, with no political ties or other influences to taint the information. This book is amazing! Well done!"

Kimberly Ohara-Borowski
Health Educator
SHAPE America National Teacher of the Year
Vice President of Health, California Association of Health, Physical Educators and Recreational Dance (CAHPERD)

"Kahn's impassioned argument for nutritionally based alternatives to traditional therapies and treatments serves as powerful inspiration for us all to seek a more holistic approach."

Amy Roby
Columnist, The Record-Courier News

"You've done well with your scientific research and current facts presentation. You have a good chapter on cancer and advocating for alternative and complementary methods."

Sonia Gaemi EdD., RD.
Founder, "Women for Cultural Wisdom" Foundation
Author, Eating Wisely for Hormonal Balance
Producer & Host, The Art of Self-Healing & International TV

"Kahn explores important issues in a thoughtful and provocative way."

Christina Cunnison
District Magnet Resource Teacher, San Mateo-Foster City

"This book is fabulous!"

Jaime Mitchell
Master of Arts, Holistic Health Education, Holistic Nutritionist
Publisher and Owner Natural Awakenings Magazine East Bay

"An important story that needs to be told."

Julia Roll
MA Teaching

"I LOVE this book!!! Excellent job of keeping the topic interesting, concise, and useful. The everyday person who does not have time to get the degree can use this book to obtain an overall view of why nutrition is important and then use it as a resource as questions arise. This is easy to read, understand and full of great information. I am not only impressed but inspired! May this be [one] of many publications you create to change the paradigm. Bravo."

Carol Wood
Family and Marriage Psychologist

"I'm glad we have people like you on this Earth to share your knowledge with the masses so hopefully one day we will be angry or motivated enough to rise up against the injustices in this world…feed people, love people and care for others!"

Rachel
A follower of A Nutrition Revolution.com

A Nutrition
Evolution

A Nutrition Evolution

Elizabeth Kahn

IngramSpark July 2019

ISBN: 978-1-7336317-2-3 (sc)
ISBN: 978-1-7336317-3-0 (hc)
ISBN: 978-1-7336317-4-7 (ebk)

Because of the dynamic nature of the Internet, any web addresses or links contained in this book may have changed since publication and may no longer be valid.

Contents

Foreword

By Jaime Mitchell

remember my pediatrician. I remember the sterile white floors, the crunchy tissue-like paper that covered the patient table, and the freezing cold temperatures of the examination room. When I was sick as a child, I distinctly remember being horrified at the thought of having to leave my house, go to the doctor, put on the patient gown and freeze while he listened to my lungs, swabbed my throat and tapped around my joints to check my reflexes. But, more than the décor, the climate and the crackling paper, I most often recall my pediatrician for his characteristic treat at the end of the visit: the lollipops.

To ease the pain and panic of any kid's trip to the doctor, my pediatrician always had a jarful of lollipops. Little white sticks topped with (undoubtedly) artificial colors, flavors, sweeteners, and corn syrup, colorfully displayed in a clear canister to entice all of us resistant children. But why wouldn't we love to visit a practitioner who made us feel better? Maybe it was because what was making us sick could have been healed with fewer trips to the doctor and more outings to the farmer's market; a little less penicillin and a few more plants.

Throughout my research at John F. Kennedy University's Master's program in holistic health education and nutrition, I became acutely aware of this country's psychological dependence on pharmaceuticals as the "only" means of healing and health. Even children are taught at a young age that if something is "wrong," only a doctor and drugs can fix it.

Elizabeth Kahn's *A Nutrition Evolution* exposes the misinformation that consumers receive from food manufacturers, drug corporations and the diet industry: information that tells us that "junk" food and diets are what we need and that drugs cure illness.

But the whistle has been blown on food, drug and diet companies in the past, which is why Elizabeth Kahn's work delves deeper. The overwhelming evidence about the corruption in our food system is only the beginning. Without workable resolutions, we are left with a dismal outlook on our health and current health-care system.

A Nutrition Evolution gives us the real "active ingredients" for nursing ourselves back to health: nutrition. When we ingest nutrients instead of popping pills—and seek nutrition guidance instead of our "doctor's orders"—we can heal ourselves and experience sustainable health.

Our health in America is on life support. We spend trillions of dollars every year on healthcare ($3 trillion in 2016), yet obesity, heart disease, autoimmune disorders, diabetes and Attention Deficit Disorder (ADD) continue to climb up the chart of concerns. We need to pull the plug on the current focus of health—from pharmaceuticals to nutrition, which is what A Nutrition Evolution does.

Elizabeth Kahn is at the forefront of a paradigm shift: a re-shifting of focus toward root causes like nutrition and education. If you are a parent, an educator, or even a policy maker, this book is a must-read for you to empower yourselves, your children, your students, and your community. Elizabeth Kahn challenges us to take health into our own hands; to realize that nutrition is the most cost-effective, most health-sustaining and most powerful anti-inflammatory, cholesterol-lowering, anti-cancer, anti-aging "product" in the market today (grocery market, that is).

When I have given nutrition talks to clients, parents and educators, I was always looking for one resource to recommend that succinctly explained food politics while providing tangible, user-friendly ideas for change. This is that guide that will now be at the top of my recommended reading list.

The time of dragging our children to the doctor whenever something is less than perfect is a thing of the past. We have the tools to be proactive health experts; to heal ourselves with the items in our refrigerator. Let's start enticing our children less with colorful lollipops at the doctor's office. It is time to introduce them to a new rainbow of colors . . . the ones you find neatly stacked around the produce section of your local grocery store.

Jaime L. Mitchell

Masters of Arts, Holistic Health Education, specialization in Holistic Nutrition

Publisher & Owner of *Natural Awakenings Magazine,* East Bay Founder of Healthy SOULutions

Introduction

"Any healthy country, like any healthy individual, should be in perpetual revolution, perpetual change."

— Jane Fonda, Activist

Since my body was healed and life was changed with nutrition, my mission has been to spread the word and help others heal naturally.

This book contains answers to questions I am asked as a nutritionist most often, including:

- "What do you think about this food, or that diet fad?"
- "Are carbohydrates bad for you?"
- "Why doesn't my doctor know more about nutrition?"
- "Why won't my insurance plan pay for nutrition consulting?"
- "What should I eat and why?"

This is not another "how to diet" book. This is a "how to understand nutrition" book. It is about *education* and making a philosophical shift in our approach to health.

We must dig deep to resolve our health and other related issues — and *that* is what *A Nutrition Evolution* does.

Since the publication of *A Nutrition Revolution* in 2011, many people have been fighting for a real-life nutrition revolution and public awareness of our extensive nutritional issues has increased. However, there is still much work to do. *A Nutrition Evolution* will help guide us on the path forward from where we are now.

Misinformation and confusion about trending diets including high-protein, high-fat, low-fat, low-carbohydrate, gluten-free, plant-based, and others are deciphered in this work. The reader will learn the fundamentals of nutrition so they can *choose* what to eat based on knowledge.

These pages contain the information needed to implement changes in our lives, grocery stores, homes, schools, doctors' offices, and voting booths, and to make the necessary shifts in our priorities and attitudes about nutrition.

Many health issues today are being caused by a poor diet, yet this fact is largely being ignored in lieu of profits. Natural and preventative solutions need a voice or voices, prepared and powerful enough to stand up to those in power to change the status quo. I am one of those voices, and that is one of the main purposes of this book, and of my work in the health and nutrition fields.

The reader will gain a true understanding of nutrition and the problems surrounding it—so we can *evolve.*

This book is dedicated to God and my Mom. Miss you, Momma: you were and still are my number one fan!

Chapter One

My Story

"Eat an apple on going to bed, and you'll keep the doctor
from earning his bread."
– English proverb

A Mystery

Years ago, I felt sick—and, like most people do when they're sick, I went to doctors for help. After several tests, I was told there was nothing wrong. I was sure *they* were wrong. I was experiencing many symptoms, including headaches, stomach aches, insomnia, moodiness, and fatigue.

The doctors did find one problem, however. One doctor said the stomach aches were due to lactose intolerance and suggested I take a pill.

Some years earlier my neighbor, who was a nutritionist, told me everyone should see a nutritionist at least once in their lives. I remembered that advice and "eenie meenie miney moed" to find one in the local phone book. I went to see her—even though my insurance paid only $20 of the $80-per-visit charge.

An Awakening

During my first visit, the nutritionist, Sonia, asked me about my symptoms and suggested I keep a food journal. Over the next few visits, we modified my diet until the right one was found, and my symptoms disappeared.

Sonia agreed with the doctor that I was lactose intolerant but also said I had other food allergies and an intestinal yeast buildup. She told me I was consuming too much white flour, too few meals and not enough vegetables. She suggested several dietary changes, recipe ideas, and a cleansing regimen. All of this helped put my body back into balance — naturally.

The difference between the philosophies of my doctor and my nutritionist can best be described by their approaches to my lactose intolerance. The doctor suggested I take a lactose pill whenever I ate dairy. The nutritionist suggested I remove the source of the problem: cow's milk.

Many of the changes my nutritionist suggested were simple and focused on eating in a more balanced way. She recommended plant-based milk, cultured dairy products that are easier to digest, more fruits and vegetables, and smaller, more frequent meals. It was more than worth the $60 out-of-pocket expense because, soon after, my symptoms were gone.

Even though drugs and doctors' visits were covered by my insurance plan, they could not help me stabilize my body *before* it broke. The nutritionist did — with only paper, pencil, and healthy food.

The money both my insurance company and I saved on more doctors' visits, tests, medication, and "special" diet food is undeniable. My private nutrition crash course cost me more immediate out-of-pocket costs, but also saved me future medical expenses and the inconvenience of developing major health issues, including hypothyroidism, diabetes, and hypoglycemia — all conditions of which I was having symptoms.

If I had not been healed through nutrition, I likely would have ended up on medications and suffered their unpleasant side effects. Instead, the "side effects" I experienced from adopting a healthier diet were increased energy, better moods, healthier hair and skin, and other health improvements I didn't even know were related.

While searching for answers, I became frustrated with the conventional medicinal approach. One of my doctors noticed my frustration and explained that they often must wait for things to break to treat them. She said the body is strong and can hold out for a while, but it will eventually break down under continued pressure. *Then* problems will show up on a test and they can begin to treat them.

While trying to handle my health issues, I bounced back and forth between doctors and the nutritionist and passed messages between them. This process worked, but I had to research it, handhold it, and pay for it. Not to mention, I was very lucky to discover this healing pathway. It would have been more efficient if:

- Practitioners worked together to solve the root of the problem
- Nutrition therapy was covered by insurance
- Nutritional healing was not a matter of luck

A History

Diabetes runs in my family. Like genes, dietary habits are also passed down. Both play an important role in diseases like diabetes, but, in our society, the impact of learned dietary habits is often ignored.

Growing up, I ate fresh, home-cooked meals every day with one parent—and doughnuts, fast food, and candy every other weekend with the other. My dad would send my three sisters and me to the doughnut store with $20 on Saturday mornings, probably to stop us from jumping on the bed and waking him up. My sisters and I went wide-eyed to Winchell's doughnut house and bought the store. This was in stark contrast to the food experience with our mother, who insisted we sit down to dinner every night and eat our vegetables.

I learned about the value of food from both of my parents—the fun from my dad and the function from my mom. But guess which side of my family has diabetes? Eating foods for fun or convenience occasionally is not a problem, but too much unhealthy food *does* cause problems—including diabetes.

My health problems began a few years after I moved out of my mother and stepfather's home. My favorite foods were Cap'n Crunch cereal, chocolate milk, and macaroni and cheese. I could not see the point of eating foods like vegetables or salads. This eventually took a toll, and, in my late twenties, I started to look and feel sick. Luckily, I discovered the negative effect my diet was having on my health and quickly altered it to feel better.

Since learning how to balance my body chemistry through nutrition, I mainly crave healthy food and no longer yearn for "junk" food. Now I can still eat an occasional doughnut—and who doesn't want to do that? But, I also crave healthy foods, including smoothies and, yes, even salads, and love the way I feel after eating them.

In quite the ironic turnaround, I now educate others about the power of nutrition and how to find a healthy *balance*. My dad's "sweet tooth" has also evolved; he now makes and sells organic honey.

Another life-altering experience that led to my nutrition career happened while watching a television news program about Attention Deficit Disorder (ADD) and diet. The show's reporters followed two children diagnosed with ADD. One boy was treated at a camp where doctors experimented with different drugs. At one point, the boy, in an apparent reaction to the drugs, stood still and stared into space while repeatedly sticking his tongue in and out. In another instance, he screamed and threw a tantrum.

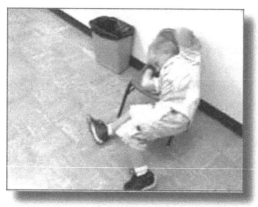

Out of Control

The news program followed a second boy to a nutrition specialist who examined his diet. Sure enough, the child tested positive for nutritional deficiencies and food allergies. After being treated with nutritional interventions his symptoms improved and he was able to get off his medications.[1]

This television program was the catalyst for a major professional life transformation for me. I was already convinced about the role of nutrition in disorders like ADD, based on my personal experiences, and I was so moved by this news program that I called a college counselor the next day to inquire about pursuing a nutrition degree. The rest, as they say, is history.

A Mission

Four and a half years of intensive study and $180,000 later, I became empowered and can now take charge of my own health and life and help others do the same. Not everyone needs a formal degree in nutrition, but everyone *should* have a basic nutrition education.

My first degree was in *clinical* nutrition, which involves a lot of chemistry, including food chemistry and biochemistry. I learned about the millions of chemical reactions occurring continuously and simultaneously in our bodies—all fueled and catalyzed by nutrition, which is the connection between our bodies and food.

Nutrition is not wizardry, but trying to find a job in prevention and natural healing was. After graduating, if I had followed the conventional path of a Registered Dietitian (RD), I would have had three basic career choices: planning hospital menus and tube feeding formulas, school district lunch menus, or providing pre-natal nutrition counseling to low-income moms. However, if a nutrition graduate like me wants to use and teach nutrition as a means of prevention to the general public, good luck! Because, there were virtually no jobs like that to be found.

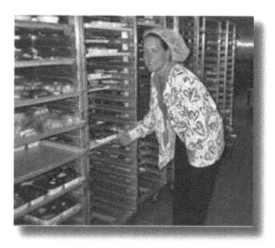

Hospital Menu Planning

So, I blazed a trail. I volunteered and worked part-time in whatever positions I could find, including not-for-profit school and community garden education programs that continually struggled for funding, and hospital and school district nutrition programs like the ones I just mentioned; and I pursued a second degree in Education.

I figured the knowledge gained from these experiences and degree would help me secure a position in one of the limited number of existing highly sought-after preventative nutrition education programs, which mainly included patient education classes offered by some healthcare providers. That was my plan at the time as, to me, it was better than striving for a career in a hospital or school district meal program with limited ability to impact change.

I ultimately earned a Health Sciences Teaching Credential and now teach Nutrition and Health Education in a public high school and maintain a private nutrition consulting practice.

As a result of hard work, determination, and faith, I finally carved out a career in education and prevention. My story this far has been a success but should not have been that difficult, and the journey isn't over.

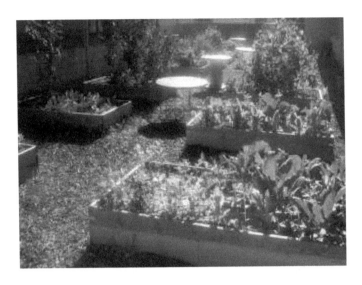

My Outdoor Classroom

The public is "hungry" for a comprehensive understanding of nutrition. Most are suffering diet-related disorders and are confused by the sea of contradictory advice and are not sure what to do or who to believe. True answers by trusted sources must be made more accessible.

Pathways to providing nutrition information include didactic programs preparing dietitians for careers geared toward *preventing* disease, increased nutrition counseling and education programs, and insurance coverage for nutrition counseling *before* diet-related diseases develop.

Nutrition information should be made more available to those who need and want it, and this should be done *early*. First, however, several obstacles must be overcome.

Chapter Two

Conventional Medicine: The Current "Go To" Solution

"It is only the inferior physician who treats the illness he was unable to prevent."
— *Chinese medical proverb*

You feel sick, so you go to the doctor — if you're lucky enough to be able to afford one these days. The response you will get from that doctor might be along the lines of:

> "I don't know what causes your problem or how to fix it, but here is a pill for your symptoms. It will probably cause side effects. If this doesn't work, we can eventually remove the malfunctioning organ and try more pills."

Or maybe something like this:

> "You have diabetes; I can prescribe diabetes medication."

> "Your thyroid is malfunctioning; I can prescribe thyroid medication."

> "You are morbidly obese; I can recommend gastric bypass surgery."

> "Your cholesterol is high; I can prescribe cholesterol medication."

The problem with these approaches is that they place an undue importance on treating *symptoms* rather than root causes. A symptom is just the body's way of saying something is wrong. Doctors don't typically look to symptoms as clues to finding their origin; instead, they try to subdue them with drugs that cause additional problems. Surgery is not ideal either, as it focuses on body parts only *after* they have broken.

Proper nutrition eliminates symptoms by addressing root causes — which are often diet related — and prevents body parts from breaking and other problems from arising due to the secondary impact of potent drugs on an already imbalanced body chemistry.

Pills vs. Plants

In medicine, when a substance is discovered that treats a condition or symptom, it is isolated, concentrated, and prescribed to the patient. Problem solved, right? Wrong. This simplistic approach not only ignores the ultimate root cause but also overlooks the complicated, delicate balance of chemicals within our bodies.

Drugs can cause side effects, which are often listed at the end of drug commercials. A commentator's voice calmly says something like: "Side effects may include rash, skin discoloration, itching, swelling, wheezing, coughing, choking, thoughts of suicide..."

Here are some *actual* possible side effects listed for a common blood-thinning medication:

> *"Side effects can include: nausea, vomiting, loss of appetite, stomach or abdominal bloating or cramps, serious bleeding, pain, swelling, discomfort, prolonged bleeding from cuts or gums, persistent nosebleeds, unusually heavy or prolonged menstrual flow, bruising, dark urine, black stools, severe headache, dizziness, nausea, vomiting, abdominal pain, yellowing of eyes or skin. This drug can cause serious (possibly fatal) complications from the dislodging of solid patches of cholesterol from blood vessel walls, which can block the blood supply to parts of the body and can cause severe tissue damage and gangrene. Other symptoms include painful red rash, dark discoloration of any body part,*

purple toe syndrome, sudden intense pain, back or muscle
pain, foot ulcers, change in the amount of urine, vision
changes, confusion, slurred speech, one-sided weakness,
rash, itching, swelling, severe dizziness, trouble breathing
and more."[1]

Historically, many foods have been used as medicine. In fact, many of today's drugs come from nature. Penicillin, the first antibiotic, came from cantaloupe mold. Herbs can be used as medicine to treat health problems. Kava root, for example, can be used to treat anxiety. St. John's Wort has been shown to alleviate depression, there are herb blends to dissipate gall stones, and herbs for many other conditions. Herbs can be used to treat just about anything pharmaceuticals can and more.

Aspirin is based on a substance found in a plant, which was, like other drugs, manipulated and concentrated. Aspirin can relieve pain and thin the blood but can also cause stomach problems and excessive bleeding. Meadowsweet—the first plant in which salicylic acid was discovered and from which aspirin was later synthesized—is an organic pain reliever and fever reducer that does not cause the harmful side effects aspirin does.[2]

We should listen to Mother Nature more instead of continually trying to improve upon her work—she has always had the answers.

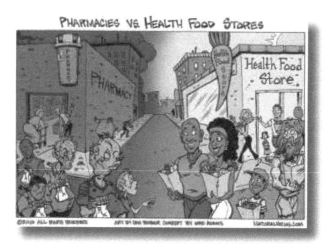

Legalize It: Medical Marijuana

The use of medical marijuana (cannabis) has been increasing in states across the U.S. as many voters have checked the box on the ballot to "legalize it." Research shows medical marijuana can treat epilepsy, chronic pain, and alleviate the side effects of chemotherapy.[3] There is speculation about, and hope for, other applications of cannabis, although more research is needed.

There has been debate about the legalization of marijuana and its use in disease treatment has been stagnated for years.

One of the main arguments used against legalization of cannabis is regarding its potentially addictive qualities. There are, of course, methods to mitigate this risk (e.g., using creams or compounds that contain low tetrahydrocannabinol [THC], the part that makes one "loopy," and high cannabidiol [CBD], which does not have the intoxicating effects of THC).

Is medical marijuana really any worse than other long-time "legal" pharmaceuticals (e.g., prescription pain killers or anti-anxiety meds)? Plants are medicine and always have been; the key is how to use them.

Happily, the secret of plant power is slowly but surely getting out. Many people believe that legalization and recognition of cannabis took so long because plants are powerful, but not as profitable as man-made substances.

Drug Money

The pharmaceutical industry, also known as "big pharma," is — year after year — one of the most profitable industries in the United States.[4] The legal drug trade brings in $450 billion a year.[5]

A billion dollars seems like a mythical number, so let's break it down: one billion dollars is equal to one-thousand million dollars. Perhaps we should think of it in terms of time: one million seconds is about 11 days. A billion seconds equates to 32 years. A trillion seconds equals 32,000 years.[6] Basically, *a lot* of U.S. dollars are being spent on prescription drugs.

Pharmaceutical companies are most likely not trying to find cures for disease or trying to prevent them, because doing so will not benefit them financially. If people get sick and stay sick, they will need more pills and the companies and shareholders will make more money — which is their ultimate goal.

The top selling drugs by disease category are:
1. Rheumatoid arthritis: $43 billion
2. Cancer: $32 billion
3. Crohn's disease: $26 billion
4. Blood thinners (heart disease): $14 billion
5. Diabetes and related issues: $11 billion[7]

All these diseases have strong links to diet.

Rheumatoid Arthritis

Rheumatoid arthritis (RA) is a condition in which the primary symptom is inflammation of the joints. Addressing food sensitivities, increasing intake of omega-3 fatty acids, and following an anti-inflammatory diet that includes plenty of whole plant foods and limits overly processed foods, can improve or reverse symptoms of RA.[8]

Since most Americans eat a diet high in inflammation-causing foods such as processed meats, potato chips, and soda, it should come as no surprise that RA is as prevalent as it is in the U.S.

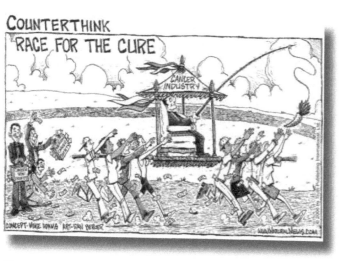

Cancer

Poor nutrition is known to be a causal factor in many types of cancer. Because the American Cancer Association (ACA) acknowledges this relationship, it recommends eating at least two and one-half cups of fruits and vegetables a day and avoiding processed foods.

There is substantial data indicating lower incidences of cancer among those who consume more plant foods and higher incidences among those who eat more animal and processed foods. Some of this data is listed in the Research chapter.

Crohn's Disease

Crohn's disease and ulcerative colitis belong to a group of conditions known as inflammatory bowel diseases (IBD), which impact the intestines. The official stance of the medical community is that there is no exact known cause, but evidence suggests a diet high in dairy, sugar, and processed foods is contributing to a higher incidence of IBD.

Despite the medical community's stance of "no known cause," the non-profit *Crohn's and Colitis Foundation* acknowledges certain foods are associated with symptoms of Crohn's.

Yogurt, white rice, and bananas have frequently been reported to reduce Crohn's symptoms, whereas spicy foods, fried foods, dairy, red meat, soda, alcohol, fatty foods, and coffee were reported to worsen symptoms.[9]

Since Crohn's and other digestive disorders are of the food processing system (intestines), it should again come as no surprise that they are related to diet and are so common these days.

Antibiotics and Probiotics

Antibiotic use has been linked to Crohn's and other chronic digestive conditions.[10] Antibiotics destroy pathogenic bacteria, but they don't discriminate; they also destroy good bacteria critical to intestinal health.

Since conventional medicine is struggling to deal with these disorders, many people are turning to natural remedies, including probiotics. Research shows probiotics can treat or prevent irritable bowel syndrome (IBS), ulcerative colitis (UC), Crohn's disease, leaky gut, and more.[11] Putting the "good guys" back in the system to solve the problem created by antibiotics just makes sense.

Blood Thinners (Heart Disease)

Diet has long been known to be an important factor in heart disease; for instance, higher incidences are linked to high-saturated fat diets. Contrarily, diets high in plant food, low in saturated fat, and high in fiber result in reduced risk.[12]

Many nutrients support and affect heart health and can even thin or thicken the blood as many medications do, but nutrients have not been studied as extensively as pharmaceuticals have in treating disease.

Can you picture a commercial advertising the health benefits of the nutrient-rich "super food" spinach—say, with happy, beautiful, healthy-looking people frolicking on a beach, such as is the script of many pharmaceutical commercials? Me either, even though that is closer to the truth than what the countless drug commercials portray.

Diabetes and Other Chronic Diseases

It is proven that consuming a healthy diet dramatically reduces incidences of diabetes, obesity, and the other prevalent illnesses. However, healthy foods are not as profitable as pharmaceuticals so there is less access to nutritional methods like nutritionists and nutrition education.

Healthcare

The lack of focus on preventative measures such as good nutrition has consequences on the U.S. health and healthcare system. As a result of this poor vision, our healthcare system is now in a quagmire.

Healthcare costs have been steadily increasing for decades. Spending rose from $348 per person in 1970 to $10,000 per person in 2016. In 2016, the U.S. spent more than $3 trillion on healthcare. By 2026, it is estimated that one out of every five U.S. dollars will be spent on healthcare. Despite this increased spending, our health outcomes remain dismal.[13]

Even though the U.S. spends nearly twice as much more per person on healthcare than any other industrialized country, we have a comparatively lower life expectancy. In addition, for the first time in U.S. history, children are projected to have a shorter lifespan than their parents.[14]

One recent study compared the cost effectiveness of healthcare in other industrialized countries including Australia, Canada, France, Germany, the Netherlands, New Zealand, Norway, Sweden, Switzerland, and the United Kingdom. The nonprofit organization that conducted the study found the American healthcare system was last or near-last in measures of health access, efficiency, and equity. The U.S. healthcare system is the most expensive in the world but performs worse than 11 other comparable nations in health outcomes. The researchers state that, although we spend a lot, the U.S. achieves neither high quality nor affordable healthcare.[13]

How did other countries fare? Of the group of 11, the United Kingdom placed first. The U.K. has a single-payer healthcare system for which many in the U.S. continue to advocate. Switzerland, which has a government-required health insurance system similar to the original U.S. Affordable Care Act (the version authorized under President Obama's administration), was number two in the rankings. However, it is important to note that, unlike the U.S., Swiss insurers are not allowed to make a profit off their basic insurance plans.[13]

The ACA is embattled, and changes continue to be proposed by those who support and those who oppose universal healthcare. So, it is not known if the U.S. will ever see the same benefits as those in the U.K., Switzerland, and others.[13]

The ongoing debates over healthcare are important, but let's also consider implementing the ultimate solution: prevention.

Medical School

Doctors do not understand nutrition because, sadly, they are not trained in it. Many receive only a two-hour nutrition lecture in medical school. Doctors *are* taught extensively about pharmaceutical and surgical solutions, however. Perhaps it is no coincidence, then, that roughly 20 percent of medical schools' yearly budgets come from the drug industry.[15]

More than half of the students graduating from medical school say their nutrition preparation was inadequate.[16] Some doctors say that what little bit of nutrition education they did receive is quite often wrong. Medical students say professors aren't talking about nutrition—and pharmaceutical companies aren't, either. The impression these future doctors get during medical school is that, if it isn't being taught, it must not be important. They *are* taught that vitamin deficiencies can cause diseases like beriberi and pellagra. However, doctors who recommend vitamins to their patients are often viewed by their counterparts as "quacks."[17]

In this country, we don't teach nutrition to doctors and do not offer it to most of the sick, yet we do provide a nutritionist to every patient in the hospital. We finally acknowledge the importance of nutrition when a patient is very ill or near death? This is too little too late. Everyone should have access to a nutritionist at the first sign of a health problem in order to keep their bodies from breaking and ending up in the hospital from diet-related illnesses.

Drug Promotion

Drug companies are strategic in selling their products and spend more money on lobbying than any other industry. In 2017 alone, lobbyists spent $25 million to encourage Congress to enact legislation to benefit the bottom lines of those they work for.[18]

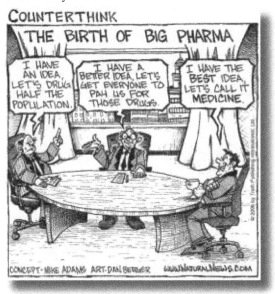

U.S. lobbyists (who are often former government officials) earn hundreds of thousands of dollars per year.[19,20] Many people working in government plan to become lobbyists after they leave their positions. It appears that many of our "public servants" are "serving" their country for personal financial gain.

In addition to promoting themselves to lawmakers, pharmaceutical companies also spend significant amounts of time and money marketing themselves to doctors and the public.

In 2012, the prescription drug industry spent over $4 billion on direct-to-consumer advertising. And it works. Doctors prescribe drugs for all types of ailments, and patients inquire about—and demand to receive—medications they've seen advertised.[21]

According to the American Medical Association Journal of Ethics, "drug advertisements... exert an undeniable influence on the way the public learns about available therapies and how patients and physicians communicate. Because advertisements' primary purpose is to sell products rather than to inform patients in an unbiased manner, reasonable oversight is essential for the public health."[21]

Some people and corporations are even being accused of "disease mongering" to maximize profits. In one paper, researchers stated that the "coming years will bear greater witness to the corporate-sponsored creation of disease."[22] Sickness should not be for profit. Instead, wellness should be.

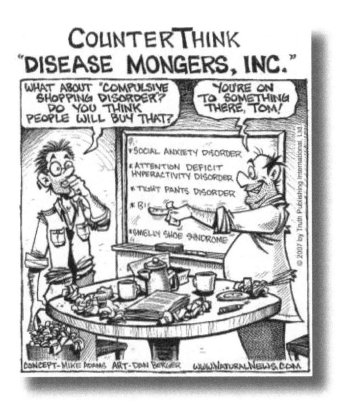

Integrated Medicine

When Western doctors and natural practitioners work together, it is called alternative, complementary, or integrated medicine. Natural practitioners include acupuncturists, chiropractors, herbalists, naturopathic doctors, nutritionists, and others who specialize in non-pharmaceutical and non-surgical interventions.

If I were in a car accident and in need of emergency surgery, I'd want to be under the care of a good surgeon. On the other hand, if I were diagnosed with cancer, I would head straight to an alternative care facility — presuming I could find and afford one.

The idea behind conventional medicine is to create "allopathy" a hostile environment for a disease in the body, so it cannot thrive. Many drugs and surgeries create a hostile environment in the body, all right. Take cancer, for instance — one of the most common diseases today. The key characteristic of cancer is that some cells in the body keep dividing; they do not know when to stop. This uncontrolled cell division is what creates tumors. Cell division is one of the most important and fundamental life processes but, in cancer, this process has gone awry.

Chemotherapy, the most common cancer treatment, is designed to kill these out-of-control cells with powerful chemicals. Patients who undergo chemotherapy feel near death because that is literally what is happening. Doctors try to stop prior to the patient actually dying, but death is the idea behind chemotherapy treatment.

There are many promising and proven natural treatments for cancer and other diseases that are not harsh or invasive, including nutritional interventions, but they are not being researched or taken seriously enough by Western medicine.[23]

The Arizona Center for Integrative Medicine, founded by natural medicine pioneer Andrew Weil, M.D., who has long been one of my inspirations, specializes in Integrative Medicine (IM) and offers re-training programs for conventional health practitioners. The center describes some of the principles of IM as follows:

- Patient and practitioner are partners in the healing process.
- All factors that influence health, wellness, and disease are taken into consideration, including body, mind, spirit, and community.
- Appropriate use of both conventional and alternative methods to facilitate the body's innate healing response.
- Effective interventions that are natural and less invasive should be used whenever possible.
- Practitioners of integrative medicine should exemplify its principles and commit themselves to self-exploration and self-development.[24]

The institute also works to push integrated medicine forward by conducting research, assisting patients in finding integrated practitioners, and educating health care practitioners from around the world in integrative medicine.

Natural medicine works to stimulate the body's own immune system and natural defenses by supporting the body so it can heal itself as it was designed to do, which is quite the opposite approach of "allopathy."

It should be the goal of all health practitioners to work together to achieve healing in the best possible way *for the patient*.

The use of natural healing methods has been increasing, including medicinal marijuana, acupuncture, and chiropractic, but we still have a long way to go.

Insurance: An Outdated Model

The main purpose of the extremely profitable insurance industry is to act as a "middle man." Logically, this is problematic, and the insurance model — and perhaps the very existence of insurance — should be reconsidered.

Nutrition has been proven to save money on healthcare costs. However, right now, nutritionists are a luxury many cannot afford. Doctors and drugs are covered by health insurance plans and preventative nutrition counseling is usually not, even though it can be at least as, or more, effective.

Nutritional interventions can not only prevent and treat disease, they save money. One study found that, if Medicare beneficiaries with high blood pressure received nutrition therapy, healthcare costs over a five-year period could be cut by an estimated $52 million.[25] If diet therapy were applied to even more diseases, the savings could be billions and even trillions of dollars.

Naturopathic Doctors (NDs) are as highly educated in the workings of the body as "Western" Medical Doctors (MDs) are, and are also trained in natural remedies including nutrition, herbal medicine, and investigating root causes such as toxins and nutrient imbalances. In spite of this, most insurance plans do not cover natural health practitioners.

I have often referred people to NDs. On each occasion, the person was healed. However, because their insurance plans wouldn't cover the visits or natural supplements, the patient paid the provider directly.

Though initially more expensive than the patient portion of a typical doctor visit, the few hundred dollars spent on natural healing was close to, or less than, the amount they would have spent on co-pays and deductibles via the conventional medical route which usually consists of multiple tests, various medications to treat symptoms, doctor visits, and eventual surgery often required because the problem was never solved. Additionally, via natural medicine, the patient was healed, which is supposed to be the goal of all healthcare approaches; and is priceless.

Another upside to this process is that the natural healthcare providers were paid directly with much less hassle and paperwork than is required when dealing with insurance. In fact, the insurance system is another "profit cycle" that works for some, although usually not the patient. We can do better.

Convenient Controversy

Two of the most profitable industries in the United States are the oil and pharmaceutical industries. This helps explain why both climate change and natural healing are controversial; because they cut into the industries' profits.

Deliberate controversy designed purely for financial gain may seem implausible, *but* some have admitted to participating in corporate smear campaigns against those who would negatively impact their companies' profits.

According to former healthcare industry executive Wendell Potter, policyholder premiums were spent to attack the movie *Sicko* which addressed the increasingly unfair and dysfunctional U.S. healthcare ystem. Potter, now a whistleblower for the insurance industry, apologized for the role he played in the industry's public relations attack campaign against the movie.

Interestingly, the front group that launched the attacks, Healthcare America, was originally a front group for the drug industry under a different name.[26] So, really, the drug and insurance industries are just defending their profits through make-believe companies and misinformation.

There are also entire websites dedicated to discrediting natural cures and practitioners. One website, "Quackwatch.com," does not call Western medicine or pharmaceuticals "quackery." Instead, they consistently apply that label to natural supplements and practitioners.

If Quackwatch were being fair, it might mention how medications often do not work and can even cause death. Quackwatch has its own credibility issues; its founder has had lawsuits filed against him, has had lawsuits he's pursued thrown out of court, and, according to a rebuttal from one of his human "targets," does not hold a valid medical license or a nutrition science degree.[27,28] I wonder who might be paying them for their "opinions."

Sometimes those with hidden agendas pose as concerned citizens. Online, these people are known as *trolls*. Trolls surf the Internet and post lies and emotionally charged comments in order to generate support for a product, company, industry, or candidate. These actions are intended to divert public attention and scrutiny away from that which they support and to create confusion and controversy which divides the public.

It is imperative to investigate sources for truthfulness and accuracy before drawing conclusions.

Conclusion

To be effective, our healthcare system must evolve from a narrow, harsh, expensive, and reactionary focus to a more inclusive, gentle, inexpensive, and preventative focus.

How do we get there? The more patients seek out, utilize, and *deman* natural methods, and question the system when it is not working, th more mainstream medicine will provide natural remedies. Natura healing will then become more common, and those currently in charge o our health will no longer be able to pretend natural solutions aren' effective or don't exist.

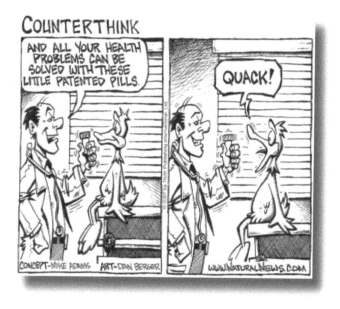

Chapter Three

Amino Acids: Building Blocks of Nutrition

"You are what you eat."
– Author unknown

Have you ever heard the saying, "You are what you eat?" Did it mean anything to you? Most people know that foods like doughnuts are bad for you and whole-grain breads are better for you, but do they know why? No—and that is why, when given the choice between whole-grain toast and a doughnut, many people would carelessly choose the latter..

A doughnut is generally more heavily processed than quality whole-grain breads. Several nutrients the body needs to function including amino acids are removed when processing foods. Amino acids comprise a portion of our DNA, which is the blueprint for life. So it is true that "you are what you eat"—and this is certainly true when it comes to amino acids in foods. Popular nutritional catch phrases must be supported with actual nutrition knowledge to have real meaning.

I first read about amino acids in *The Vitamin Bible,* which details nutrients such as amino acids and their functions.[1] *The Vitamin Bible* is what first convinced me of the power of nutrition. Amino acids are the foundations of life and were also, ironically enough, the foundation of *my* new life. Reading about amino acids started me on a path that eventually led me to become a nutritionist.

Amino acids are the building blocks of protein. They create energy by turning food into fuel. They also act as antioxidants, detoxifying our bodies.

Amino acids send messages, catalyze chemical reactions, and form molecules such as heme, a component of blood, which transports oxygen and iron and distributes them to the cells in our bodies.

There are approximately 28 commonly known amino acids. 80 percent can be made in the body. However, the rest must be obtained through the diet. The amino acids the body cannot produce are called "essential" amino acids. These include histidine, isoleucine, leucine, lysine, methionine, phenylalanine, threonine, tryptophan, and valine. "Non-essential" amino acids include alanine, arginine, asparagine, aspartic acid, citrulline, cysteine, cystine, gamma-amino butyric acid, glutamic acid, glutamine, glycine, ornithine, proline, serine, taurine, and tyrosine. Amino acids are found in protein-rich foods such as meat, milk, fish, soy, whole grains, beans, nuts, and seeds.[2]

When we do not get the right amount of amino acids, our bodies can break down. Imbalances of these nutrients have been implicated in countless health problems, including depression, schizophrenia, ADD, Alzheimer's, autism, dementia, epilepsy, chronic fatigue syndrome, erectile dysfunction, bipolar syndrome, excess body fat, tumor growth, and multiple sclerosis.[1,2,3,4]

A basic knowledge of amino acids and other nutrients is essential to understanding nutrition. Here are a few examples of amino acids and what they do and why they are so important. The amino acids not listed each have different roles, and are also critically important.

Histidine

- Used for tissue repair and nerve cell protection. Removes heavy metals from the system. Lowers blood pressure and may help prevent AIDS.
- May aid sexual functioning and arousal.
- Symptoms of imbalance include stress, anxiety, schizophrenia, rheumatoid arthritis, and nerve deafness. Imbalances may intensify manic or bipolar symptoms and can contribute to

diseases such as Alzheimer's, Parkinson's and diabetes.

- Food sources include rice, rye, and wheat.[1,2]

Phenylalanine

- Converted into tyrosine, dopamine, and norepinephrine, which promote alertness; is a painkiller, antidepressant, appetite suppressant, aids in memory and learning, and can be used to treat arthritis, depression, menstrual cramps, migraines, obesity, Parkinson's disease, and schizophrenia.
- Symptoms of imbalance include increased blood pressure and moodiness; and interference with serotonin, which affects mood, sleep, and appetite.
- Food sources include beans, beef, chicken, soy, and spirulina or seaweed. It is found naturally in breast milk and in the manufactured food product aspartame. Phenylalanine is added to many foods including sodas and chewing gum.[1,2]

Tryptophan

- A building block of serotonin, melatonin, and niacin; can aid in sleep; is a calming agent and antidepressant; can treat epilepsy; stabilizes moods; can relieve migraine headaches and nicotine withdrawal.
- Tryptophan is called the natural alternative to Prozac. Psychiatrists sometimes prescribe tryptophan to those who do not respond to antidepressant drug treatments.
- Symptoms of imbalance include pellagra, coronary artery spasms, depression, and insomnia.
- Food sources include bananas, brown rice, corn, dairy products, eggs, fish, mushrooms, poultry, and red meat.[1,2,5]

Tyrosine

- A precursor to norepinephrine and dopamine; is a mood elevator; contributes to the production of morphine in the body; can treat medication-resistant depression, anxiety, cocaine and other drug addiction/withdrawal, chronic fatigue syndrome, narcolepsy, low sex drive, allergies, headaches and Parkinson's disease.

- Symptoms of imbalance include depression, low blood pressure, low body temperature (cold feet and hands), hypothyroidism, and restless leg syndrome.
- Food sources include almonds, avocados, bananas, corn, dairy products, fish, lima beans, mushrooms, poultry, and soy. Tyrosine is being added to many food products, including energy drinks.[1,2]

Nutrients and Disease

Pellagra, pictured below, is a skin disease caused by a tryptophan deficiency. This disease is a good example of the benefits of nutrients and of man's often confusing search for them. In 1918, a scientist hired to find a cure to the pellagra epidemic that had killed 11 thousand people in the southern U.S. discovered that a high-quality protein diet could cure the condition. Despite this discovery, pellagra continued to be fatal for many.

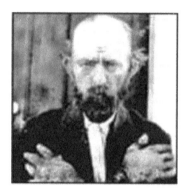

Pellagra

Pellagra killed more than 27,000 people in the years following the discovery about the relationship between diet and the disease. The problem was that B-complex vitamins were not isolated in a lab until 1930. Because scientists did not know tryptophan was a precursor to vitamin B3, they ignored the relationship between diet and pellagra. They simply could not "connect the dots."[5]

Many substances and chemical pathways are still yet to be discovered.

Therefore, we are still missing some "dots" and, no doubt, still ignoring what works because we haven't isolated all of the reasons for it in a lab yet.

Nutrients and Synergy

The chemicals in our bodies work together in an intricate balance called "synergy," a word derived from the Greek word "synergos" which means "working together." Amino acids and other nutrients work together and share pathways in our bodies. Nutrients must be in balance or they can be ineffective—either because they have to compete with each other or are missing a necessary counterpart needed to function.

For example, if a weightlifter takes the amino acid arginine to gain muscle mass, his body's ability to absorb lysine, another amino acid, will be reduced. This is because these two amino acids share the same transport systems.[6] This situation is analogous to two people needing a taxi to get to work but there is only one—and it only has one seat. As a result, only one person at a time can ride. The one left behind *may* find another way to get where they are going, but it won't be as timely or effective.

Every imbalance creates a chain reaction. This taxi analogy can be applied to many nutrients in the body. Imagine all the potential problems caused by a single nutrient imbalance—which causes a backup on one end because too many nutrients are waiting for a ride and a shortage of workers on the other end because too few nutrients arrived to work. The excessive amounts of workers waiting for a ride can overfill the waiting area and cause a wall to fall over *and* the workers' jobs at the intended destination will not get done.

Additional nutrients, like innocent bystanders, may also get stuck in the backup or have trouble doing their job because the nutrients they relied on didn't show up for work, and on and on. This cumulative effect will often cause something along one of the affected areas or "chains" to break. In the meantime, the body will probably not function as it should, and the host may feel lethargic or sick. The longer an imbalance continues, the more likely a break will occur. This describes one of the many ways the body can malfunction due to nutrient imbalances and why synergy and balance are so critically important. This also explains why we should consider the whole-grain bread over the doughnut (and many other food choices) more thoughtfully and more often.

Balanced, healthy diets are beneficial because nutrients work synergistically and the types and amounts matter. We know this to be true, yet we persist on a path of imbalance and illness due to the ingredients of ignorance and profits in a recipe for disaster.

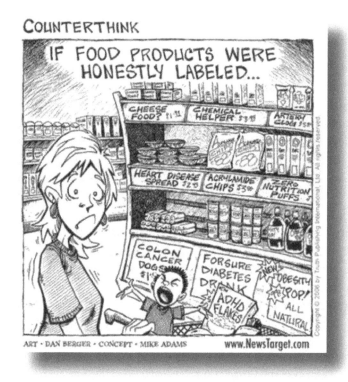

Amino acids are added to manufactured foods including energy drinks, diet soda, and gum, and are *removed* when processing whole foods. For example, amino acids are removed when making white flour which is one of the most popular food products on the market today.

There has recently been a public outcry against eating grains and gluten, the ingredient some grains contain. This is because of what food manufacturers have done to the otherwise "innocent" whole-wheat grain. Let's look at what happens when they "refine" or overly "process" whole wheat grain.

A grain of whole-wheat has three main parts: the bran, germ, and endosperm.

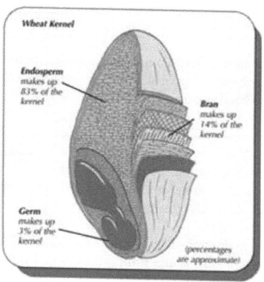

Whole-Wheat Grain

The parts of the whole-wheat grain with the most amino acids are the bran and germ which are the parts removed when making white flour. All that is left in white flour is the endosperm which not only has fewer amino acids, but is also full of the protein gluten. Food manufacturers love gluten because it is extremely pliable *and* tasty. However, many people are developing gluten sensitivities as a result of consuming too much white flour.

Protein quality depends on all the essential amino acids being present in the right amounts, and, in complete proteins, they are. According to a measurement by The Institute of Medicine (IOM), a complete protein has a score of 100.[7] Here is a Report Card—based on numeric scores—for the individual parts of a grain of wheat.

Report Card — Wheat Grain	
Grain Component	Protein Quality
Germ	A
Bran	C
Endosperm	F

White flour fails the amino acid quality test, among others. The Processed Food chapter explores more precisely which nutrients, including amino acids, are removed when processing foods such as white flour.

Amino acid imbalances cause many health issues, including erectile dysfunction (ED).[3,4] You may not know this, but I bet you know there are various medications available to treat ED. The annual ED drug market is estimated to be over $3 billion, and a bottle of ED pills costs about $700. Therefore, manufacturers advertise them, *a lot*.[8,9]

Whole foods, rich in balanced amounts of amino acids, are far less profitable, so there is not as much motivation to sell them. Got quinoa? Did you know quinoa is an easy-to-cook, gluten-free, delicious whole-grain that is a complete protein that may help with ED and other disorders? No? Perhaps we need some advertisements for that.

Conclusion

Our advanced society has made many beneficial discoveries. However, when it comes to our health, Mother Nature still knows best. So, until we know more than she does, we should listen to her wisdom, combined with our own, and consume more whole foods with naturally synergistic amounts of nutrients like amino acids. By doing so, countless lives will be improved and *saved*.

Chapter Four

Micronutrients: "Worker Bees"

"The wise man should consider that health is the greatest of human blessings. Let food be your medicine."
— Hippocrates

Have you ever heard the statement, "Get your vitamins?"

Micronutrients are nutrients the body needs in small amounts. These include vitamins and minerals which the body needs in order to grow, develop, function, and heal itself from illness and injury. When the body does not get the right amount of any micronutrient, it will not function properly and can break.

We all know we are supposed to eat healthy and get plenty of vitamins and minerals, but many of us don't do it because we don't know which ones we need, what foods to find them in, or *why* we need them. Again, I will use the doughnut example.

How many vitamins do you think are in a doughnut? Not many. The more people know, the more likely they are to make a healthier choice more often, don't you agree? Let's examine the importance of what these nutrients do and then, maybe, we will care a bit more and not *always* choose the doughnut over a more nutritious choice.

Vitamins

There are 13 vitamins your body needs that it cannot produce — vitamins A, C, D, E, K, and the B vitamins including biotin, niacin, pantothenic acid, riboflavin, thiamine, vitamin B-6, B-9 (folate or folic acid) and B-12. Each vitamin has a specific job.[1]

Vitamin imbalances are implicated in several health issues, including ADD, heart disease, erectile dysfunction, depression, night blindness, skin disorders, chronic fatigue, obesity, diabetes, high cholesterol, blood pressure issues, and blood thinness or thickness. Here are details about the functions of a few vitamins and foods that contain them:

Vitamin A

- Plays an important role in vision, growth, reproduction, and immune function.
- Symptoms of imbalance include night blindness, dry eye syndrome, poor growth, dry skin, lowered immunity, headaches, vomiting, hair loss, liver damage, skin problems, birth defects, and bone pain.
- Food sources include broccoli, carrots, fish, fortified milk, leafy greens, liver, peaches, and sweet potatoes.[2]

Vitamin B1/Thiamin

- Enhances circulation; assists in blood formation, carbohydrate metabolism, and hydrochloric acid formation (which assists in digestion); optimizes cognitive activity and brain function; has a positive effect on energy, growth, appetite, and learning capacity; acts as an antioxidant; and contributes to protecting the body from the degenerative effects of aging, alcohol consumption, and smoking.
- Symptoms of imbalance include beriberi (a nervous system disease), constipation, edema, an enlarged liver, fatigue, forgetfulness, gastrointestinal disturbances, heart changes, irritability, labored breathing, loss of appetite, muscle atrophy, nervousness, numbness of the hands and feet, pain and sensitivity, poor coordination, tingling sensations, weak and sore muscles, general weakness, and severe weight loss.
- Food sources include brown rice, eggs, fish, legumes, liver, peanuts, peas, pork, poultry, and whole grains.[3]

Vitamin B12/Methylcobalamin

- Active in growth and protection of the nervous system. May help prevent and slow progression of Parkinson's disease, reverse symptoms of Bell's palsy, and shows promise of treating multiple sclerosis and other neurological diseases. Is involved in cardiovascular function, protein synthesis and building, and may produce nerve regeneration. Needed to prevent anemia, and is involved in sleep, digestion, and learning.
- Deficiencies can be caused by malabsorption, common in older individuals and those with digestive disorders. Deficiencies can cause abnormal gait, bone loss, chronic fatigue, constipation, digestive disorders, dizziness, drowsiness, enlargement of the liver, eye disorders, hallucinations, headaches (including migraines), inflammation of the tongue, irritability, labored breathing, memory loss, moodiness, nervousness, neurological damage, palpitations, pernicious anemia, ringing in the ears, and spinal cord degeneration.
- Food sources include brewer's yeast, dairy products, eggs, fish, fortified foods including cereals and plant milks (such as almond, rice, and soy), meat, sea vegetables (such as dulse, kelp, kombu, and nori), and soybeans.[4]

Vitamin C/Ascorbic Acid

- An antioxidant required for tissue growth and repair, adrenal gland function, and healthy gums; aids in formation of anti-stress hormones; helps metabolize folic acid, tyrosine, and phenylalanine; protects against pollution and infection; helps prevent cancer; enhances immunity; increases the absorption of iron; may reduce cholesterol levels and high blood pressure and prevent atherosclerosis; helps with formation of collagen; protects against blood clotting and bruising; and promotes healing of wounds and burns.
- Symptoms of imbalance include scurvy (characterized by poor wound healing), soft and spongy bleeding gums, edema, extreme weakness, hemorrhages under the skin, gums that bleed when brushing teeth, increased susceptibility to infection, joint

pains, lack of energy, poor digestion, prolonged healing time, a tendency to bruise easily, and tooth loss.

- Food sources include asparagus, avocados, cantaloupe, grapefruit, lemons, onions, oranges, persimmons, pineapple, spinach, and strawberries.[3]

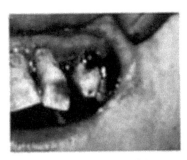

Teeth Showing Effects of Scurvy

Vitamin D

- Necessary for the absorption of calcium and phosphorus by the intestinal tract, for growth and for tooth and bone formation, normal blood clotting, thyroid function, regulation of the heartbeat, and immunity. Protects against muscle weakness, osteoporosis, and hypocalcemia.
- Symptoms of imbalance include rickets (softening and weakening of bones in children), loss of appetite, a burning sensation in the mouth and throat, diarrhea, insomnia, visual problems, and weight loss.

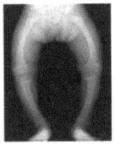

A Child's Legs Showing Effects of Rickets

- Food sources include dairy products, eggs, fish liver oils, fatty saltwater fish, liver, oatmeal, and sweet potatoes. Exposure to sunlight (without sunblock) is also a good source of vitamin D.[3]

Minerals

Minerals come from the earth and are absorbed by plants and water and then by the animals that consume them. The minerals your body needs include calcium, chloride, chromium, copper, fluoride, iodine, iron, magnesium, manganese, molybdenum, phosphorus, potassium, selenium, sodium, and zinc. Some minerals, such as lead, are not needed and can be toxic.

Vital minerals perform many important functions such as forming and maintaining healthy bones and skin and for blood flow and oxygen exchange. Mineral imbalances can cause many health problems including ADD, autism, depression, and fatigue.[4]

Calcium

- Essential for formation and maintenance of bone and plays a vital role in nerve transmission, muscle contraction, blood pressure regulation, and the release of hormones.
- Symptoms of imbalance include loss of bone mass, increased risk of osteoporosis, bone fractures, and kidney stones.
- Food sources include broccoli, Chinese cabbage, dairy products, kale, legumes, and sardines.[2]

Iron

- Aids in producing hemoglobin which is an essential cofactor for enzymes that are involved in numerous cellular processes, is important for growth, delivery of oxygen to red blood cells, a healthy immune system, and energy production.
- Symptoms of imbalance include anemia, fatigue, decreased resistance to infection, changes in behavior, decreased work capacity, decreased resistance to infection, adverse pregnancy

outcomes, inability to adapt to cold weather, pica (desire to eat non-food substances), increased risk of lead poisoning, impaired cognitive ability, weakness, and lethargy. Note: Iron works with zinc, copper, manganese and molybdenum, and its effectiveness is dependent on the proper balance of each of these nutrients.

- Food sources include eggs, fish, green leafy vegetables, kidney beans, liver, raisins, red meat and whole grains.[2,3]

Potassium

- Important for a healthy nervous system and regular heart rhythm; helps prevent stroke; aids in proper muscle contraction, water balance, and maintaining stable blood pressure; sends electro-chemical impulses; and regulates transfer of nutrients in the body.
- Symptoms of imbalance include dry skin, acne, chills, cognitive impairment, constipation, depression, diarrhea, lowered reflex function, edema, nervousness, thirst, glucose intolerance, irregular heartbeat, insomnia, high cholesterol, low blood pressure, muscular fatigue, headaches, nausea, vomiting, growth impairment, respiratory distress, salt retention, and protein in the urine. The function of potassium can decrease with age, and this may account for some of the circulatory damage, weakness, and lethargy experienced by older people.
- Food sources include dairy products, fish, fruit, legumes, meat, poultry, vegetables, and whole grains.[3]

Sodium

- Necessary for maintaining proper blood pH and water balance and the proper functioning of the stomach, muscles, and nerves.
- Symptoms of imbalance include abdominal cramps, anorexia, confusion, dehydration, depression, dizziness, fatigue, flatulence, headache, heart palpitations, lethargy, muscular weakness, memory impairment, poor coordination, recurrent infections, seizures, and weight loss. A proper balance of sodium and potassium is necessary in the body, and a high intake of sodium can cause a potassium deficiency.

- Virtually all foods contain some sodium. Most of us get enough, and some may get too much, but deficiencies do occur—especially when taking certain medications. More natural sources of sodium such as sea salt are best.[3]

Supplements: Should I or Shouldn't I?

Since whole food contains synergistic amounts of nutrients, it is preferable to get the nutrients we need through food. However, for many people, this can be a challenge. Therefore, taking a quality, plant-based supplement can be beneficial for some people, but there are caveats.

Spot-taking nutrients (e.g., taking one or two nutrients at a time) can be problematic as nutrients work synergistically, as mentioned earlier.

There are many poor-quality supplements on the market that do not contain what they claim to, are synthetic (man-made), or have sugar or chemicals added to them.

A qualified natural health practitioner can advise one about nutrients, amounts, and brands of supplements to take. This can save time and money and provide the best chance to gain the optimal health benefits of supplements.

Conclusion

There are many different vitamins and minerals, and each plays a unique and vital role in the millions of chemical reactions happening in the human body. When one nutrient is missing or in excess, disruption occurs in the natural organic pathways the body was meant to facilitate. "Playing" with food and over-eating foods with imbalanced amounts of nutrients confuses the system and causes malfunctions in the body—and this is mainly why consuming whole foods is ideal.

The medical community and public were once oblivious to the fact that nutrient deficiencies were behind conditions such as scurvy and rickets. However, many public health problems still exist today, though often more subtle and chronic, due to nutrient imbalances and people are still suffering needlessly. Therefore, continuing to ignore nutrition's role in disease is plain *negligence*.

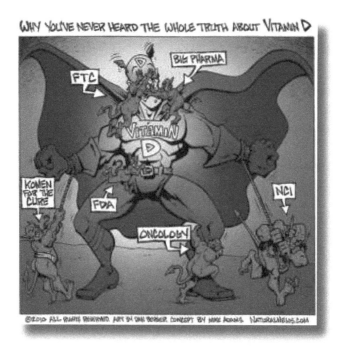

Chapter Five

Macronutrients: Nuts and Bolts

"To eat is a necessity, but to eat intelligently is an art."
— *Francois de La Rochefoucauld*

Macronutrients are nutrients needed by the body in large amounts, and include carbohydrates, protein, fat, water, and air. As is the case with all other nutrients, macronutrient imbalances cause problems in the body. Many macronutrients including fat, protein, and carbohydrates, are being talked about quite a bit as of late. Therefore, let's shed some light on the controversy and confusion surrounding nutrition's "big" nutrients.

Let's talk about that doughnut again first, shall we? I really don't mean to pick on the yummy food product, but it is now a theme. As has been discussed previously, the doughnut lacks nutrients like amino acids, vitamins, and minerals. It does have a lot of some nutrients however, including carbohydrates, the bad ones, and fat, which we should limit. The doughnut is just one example of the many nutritionally flawed foods a lot of people are overeating. Without further ado, let's dive into macronutrients more deeply to better understand them and make more empowered and motivated choices about them.

Carbohydrates

One of the most popular recent diet fads is a low-carbohydrate diet. The main problem with that is carbohydrates are a primary source of fuel for the body. Carbohydrates are not "the enemy." In fact, no single nutrient or food group is "the enemy," although a solid argument could be made for "junk" food. Rather, *imbalance* is the enemy. Overdoing anything — fat, salt, sugar, protein, carbohydrates, or heavily processed foods — is the real problem.

So, let's take a moment to give poor, misunderstood carbs some credit. Besides being a major source of energy for the body, and having many other health benefits, carbohydrates aid digestion and have a mild tranquilizing effect on the brain.

Considering that plants are the main source of carbohydrates, it is easy to understand why a "no" or "low-carb" diet is a pretty impractical idea. What we need to understand is how to consume a variety of foods including carbohydrates in *healthy* ways.

Simple Carbohydrates

Carbohydrates come in two forms: simple and complex. They are made up of chains of sugar molecules. The longer the chain, the more complex the carbohydrate, and the slower it is digested. The shorter the chain, the faster it is digested.

Simple carbohydrates cause a quick spike in blood sugar because they break down faster than complex carbs. Repeating that cycle at high rates is hard on the pancreas and other organs and contributes to various health problems including diabetes.

The main issue with carbohydrates is that many people are eating too many simple carbohydrates—usually in the form of processed foods—and not enough of the "good" carbohydrates found in whole foods.

Simple carbs are found in foods such as fruit juices, high-fructose corn syrup, milk, soda, sugar, white flour, and white rice. Overconsumption of simple carbs, especially those found in refined foods, can lead to many problems, including diabetes, hypoglycemia and obesity.

Complex Carbohydrates

Complex carbs are often referred to as the "good carbs." Fiber is a complex carbohydrate. Complex carbohydrates are found in foods such as fruits, vegetables, beans, and whole grains. These are the ones we *should* be eating plenty of.

Fiber is the body's natural cleanser and helps "clean our pipes" or intestines. Fiber increases turnover of toxins and other waste products by changing the consistency of the "garbage" for a more efficient elimination. Clean pipes allow nutrients to cross through intestinal walls and enter the bloodstream to be utilized for many important bodily processes.

Consuming sufficient amounts of fiber lowers the risk of colon cancer, helps lower blood cholesterol levels, and reduces the risk of heart disease.

Too much fiber, however, can interfere with nutrient absorption, although, that is not a problem for most people. The typical American diet relies heavily on processed foods, animal products, and sugary drinks that contain little to no fiber.

Symptoms of a carbohydrate deficiency include digestion and kidney problems, and fatigue.

Recommendations

It is recommended that between 45 to 65 percent of a person's total daily calories come from carbohydrates, which is 900 to 1,300 calories for a 2,000-calorie-per-day diet, or approximately 25 grams for an adult female and 38 grams for an adult male. The exact recommended amounts depend on the individual's age, activity level, and gender.

Protein

Proteins are chains of amino acids. They make up the greatest portion of our body weight after water and are a part of every living cell. Protein is needed for growth and development and helps maintain water balance and pH (a measure of acidity and alkalinity in the body). Proteins are found in muscles, ligaments, tendons, organs, glands, hair, nails, and vital body fluids. The hormones and enzymes that catalyze and regulate all bodily processes are proteins.[1] Protein can be found in animal *and* plant foods.

Protein excesses can cause dehydration, digestive problems, high cholesterol, increased cancer risk, kidney issues, and weight gain. Protein deficiencies can cause conditions such as edema, kwashiorkor, malnutrition, and muscle loss.

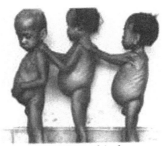
Kwashiorkor

Recommendations

It is recommended that between 10 to 35 percent of a person's total daily calories come from protein, which is 200 to 700 calories for a 2,000-calorie diet, or approximately 46 grams a day for adult women and 56 grams for adult men.

Most American's consume *too much* protein, often in the form of unhealthy, fatty, and processed meats. Protein will be discussed further in the Healthy Eating chapter.

Fat

The body and brain need fat. Fat performs many important functions:

- Provides insulation for the body
- Provides cushion for the organs
- Protects against temperature changes
- Helps with nerve transmission and muscle contraction
- Aids in memory[3]
- Source of energy
- Protects against inflammation
- Helps absorb some vitamins and minerals
- Essential for blood clotting
- Vital exterior for each cell[4]

Some argue that fat has been overly vilified. However, a diet full of bacon and other fatty, processed meats — which is what some modern-day diet advocates recommend — is not the answer. This will only create *new* imbalances and cause *new* problems. The key is to learn how to achieve a healthy balance of *all* the nutrients.

Saturated Fat

Saturated fat has as many hydrogen bonds attached to it as is possible — hence the name "saturated." In other words, it is "full" of hydrogen atoms.

Excessive consumption of saturated fat has been linked to obesity, heart disease, heart attacks, strokes, and other health issues.

The health risks associated with high-saturated-fat diets probably have as much or more to do with a lack of consumption of nutritious plant foods (which is typical in these diets) as it does with consuming saturated fat itself. Therefore, whole plant foods are more likely the real "heroes," and saturated fats are probably neither villain *nor* hero, but just need to be consumed in moderation.

Saturated fats are found primarily in animal products such as dairy products, eggs, and meat, but can also be found in some plant foods such as coconut and palm kernel oils.

Recommendations

The recommended daily limit for saturated fat is five to 10 percent of total daily calories, which is 100 to 200 calories or 11 to 22 grams, for a 2,000-calorie-per-day diet. Most Americans exceed these amounts.[5,6]

A vast amount of research clearly proves we need fat; however, it has not been proven that we *need* saturated fat.

Trans fats

Trans fats, which are mainly found in processed foods, should be avoided altogether. Trans fats are also covered in the Processed Food chapter.

Unsaturated Fats

Unsaturated fats, which are considered the healthy fats, include poly-unsaturated and mono-unsaturated fats.

Mono means "one." Mono-unsaturated fats have one empty space where a hydrogen atom would be present in a saturated fat molecule. Mono-unsaturated fats can be found in nuts, avocados, canola oil, olive oil, safflower oil (high oleic), sunflower oil, peanut oil, butter, and sesame oil.

The Mediterranean Diet originated from the low rates of heart disease found among populations that consumed high amounts of mono-unsaturated fats (e.g., olive oil) vs. those that consumed high amounts of saturated fats (e.g., most animal products).

Poly means "many." Poly-unsaturated means there are many empty spaces where a hydrogen atom would be in a saturated fat molecule. Poly-unsaturated fats include the omega-3 and omega-6 fatty acids, and the "essential fat" linoleic acid, which is a fat the body needs but cannot make, so must be obtained through diet.

Some of the many health benefits of unsaturated fats include preventing and treating diseases including heart disease, memory problems such as dementia, and inflammatory disorders including rheumatoid arthritis. Unsaturated fats are also involved in muscle movement, building cell membranes, blood clotting, and covering nerves.[4]

Good sources of poly-unsaturated fats include walnuts, sunflower seeds, flax seeds, and fish such as salmon, mackerel, herring, albacore tuna, and trout. Recommendations are listed at the end of this section.

Cholesterol

Cholesterol is found in animal products including meat, eggs, shellfish, and butter. Cholesterol is important for cell structure, digestion, absorption, and making hormones. Most people consume too much cholesterol. The human body can make its own, so there is no dietary requirement for cholesterol.

Recommendations

Currently, there are no exact recommendations for cholesterol because those tasked with determining the recommended amounts found insufficient data that proved cholesterol *itself* causes health problems. However, foods that contain cholesterol usually are high in saturated and trans fats, and since we do not need dietary cholesterol, cholesterol should still be limited.[7]

The most recent recommended limits for cholesterol were 200 milligrams (mg) for anyone at risk for heart disease, and 300 mg a day for everyone else. However, most American men eat about 350 mg and women average about 240 mg a day.[6]

Digging Deeper into Fatty Foods

Many people think they need to eliminate entire groups of foods or food products including fatty ones, but this is not always true. The truth is that knowledge about the nutritional content of foods can create *options*.

For example, there are many types of cheeses and nutritional variations among them. Most cheese is made from cow or goat milk; however, there are also many plant-based cheeses available on the market today that are derived from various sources including cashews, almonds, and soy.

Let's compare the saturated fat and cholesterol content of a few cheeses. The following chart examines the popular cow's milk cheeses: cheddar, Swiss, mozzarella, and one plant-based (soy) cheese.

Cheese Type	Saturated Fat (Grams)	Cholesterol (Milligrams)
Cheddar	14	70
Swiss	12	61
Mozzarella	8	44
Soy	1	0

Note: Amounts are based on ½-cup servings.[8]

As you can see, mozzarella has less saturated fat and cholesterol than cheddar or Swiss, and plant-based cheese has even less or none. So, as this example illustrates, healthy eating does not necessarily mean avoidance, but it does mean *awareness*.

Overall Fat Recommendations

Recommendations are approximately 20 to 35 percent of daily calories come from fat (mainly unsaturated fat) which is 400 to 700 calories or 44 to 78 grams, for a 2,000-calorie-per-day diet.[5,6]

Water

Water provides a foundation for and participates in chemical reactions, regulates body temperature, removes waste products, transports nutrients, maintains acid-base balance, and processes vitamins. Water affects every action within the body, and therefore a water imbalance can impair just about any bodily function.

Symptoms of a water deficiency in the body include excess body fat, headaches, poor muscle tone, digestive problems, muscle soreness, stomach aches, fatigue, water retention, and poor functioning of organs.

Conversely, proper hydration can slow the aging process; prevent and improve health conditions including arthritis, diabetes, digestive problems, glaucoma, kidney stones, and obesity.

Unfortunately, water can be unhealthy *and* unsafe. Many water companies do not meet the basic requirements of the Environmental Protection Agency (EPA) for safe levels of toxic substances in our water including arsenic, copper, iron, radon, lead, fluoride, bacteria, pesticides, and heavy metals. Water can also contain chemicals not yet being tested for. It is estimated that over 60 million people in the U.S. are drinking water contaminated by industrial waste dumping, farming practices, and deteriorating water systems.[9] Tap water quality can be checked at the Environmental Working Group website: EWG.org.

Many people turn to water in plastic bottles to ensure they are consuming safe water. The quality and benefits of bottled water are often questionable however, and the material in which water is packaged has created a massive environmental issue. Every year, 300 million tons of plastic are produced globally, half of which is single-use plastic including water bottles and food packaging. The plastic ends up in the landfills which are overfilled, or end up in the waterways. In fact, more than eight million tons of plastic are dumped into our oceans every year.[10]

Alkaline Water

Pure water has a neutral pH value of 7. More basic or "alkaline" water has a higher pH value and is less acidic than pure water. The Western Diet is very acidic and can cause health problems; so, many people are turning to alkaline water to help balance this out. Alkaline water has been shown to improve health conditions such as arthritis and digestion problems. I consume alkaline water (9.5 pH) and have experienced many health benefits as a result, including improved digestion and healthier skin.

Recommendations

Most people should consume at least eight 8-ounce glasses of quality water a day.[11] I recommend purchasing from a reputable water supplier or using a good water filter and using reusable water bottles rather than single-use plastic bottles.

Try this refreshing concoction as a fun and enjoyable way to drink more water. This is also a great soda replacer!

Beth's Healthy Spritzer
Ingredients:
4 ounces 100% fruit juice
4 ounces carbonated water
½ cup ice
Directions: Pour all ingredients into glass and enjoy!

Air

Air is a macronutrient that is critical to life. Oxygen is the most powerful substance in the body and provides life to all cells. Animals and plants have a symbiotic relationship with air. Humans breathe in, or inhale, (O_2) and breathe out, or exhale, carbon dioxide (CO_2), whereas plants inhale CO_2 and exhale O_2.

However, not all air is good for you. A 2010 American Lung Association "State of the Air" report found that roughly 58 percent of the population suffers from exposure to air pollution levels that are often too dangerous to breathe. Over time, taking in these particles—mainly pollution from factories and cars—may increase the risk of asthma, lung damage, and death.[12]

Many toxic household and personal products are also being inhaled. These include air fresheners, hair spray, and cleaning products. These substances affect the natural respiratory function, other body processes, and can adversely affect our health.

A Toxic Mix

These days, toxins are everywhere. We eat, drink, breathe, and apply an array of destructive man-made chemicals. To exacerbate these problems, most people don't consume enough healthy foods that naturally purge these unnatural substances from the body. Therefore, we must more carefully contemplate the toxins in our environment *and* consume more whole plant foods and quality water that help cleanse our bodies of these unhealthy "invaders."

Conclusion

These chapters were written to illustrate the fundamentals and importance of nutrition without overwhelming the reader with too much technical information or diving too deeply into any one topic. Some nutritional concepts are complex and, as a result, nutrition information is being misrepresented and misunderstood. This work is meant to provide a foundation from which to understand nutrition on a deep enough level for the lay person to navigate the sea of conflicting and confusing nutrition information and create a healthy, sustainable diet that works for them.

Chapter Six

Healthy Eating: Putting the Pieces Together

"Eat food. Not too much. Mostly plants."
— Michael Pollan

"Eat a healthy diet."

"Lose weight."

Have you heard these recommendations from your doctor or someone else? What do these statements mean? How would one accomplish these tasks? By avoiding carbohydrates, red meat, sugar, salt, fat, or drinking weight-loss shakes for most meals? Eating salad (with no dressing), a baked skinless chicken breast, and steamed vegetables? Not eating fried food, fast food, or dessert ever again?

A "healthy diet" is often recommended to achieve health goals such as losing weight, reversing or relieving symptoms of diabetes, high blood pressure, or obesity. However, this advice is often insufficient and difficult to know how to follow.

By the end of this chapter, you will have a better understanding of what a *sustainable* healthy diet means—which usually leads to many health benefits including achieving and maintaining a healthy weight.

Healthy eating means eating foods with nutrients the body needs to function optimally. Food is meant to provide energy, sustain, and *heal* us. Contrary to many diet philosophies out there, we need to *eat* a variety of food. Healthy eating can be fun and satisfying. It can mean eating the foods we love including the so-called "bad stuff" —just not a lot of it. Many people do not know what healthy eating means because they do not fundamentally *understand* nutrition.

I have counseled many people on how to "eat a healthy diet" by incorporating their personal preferences into an eating plan that works for them and their lifestyle.

My students and clients find nutrition knowledge empowering—and that leads to them developing a healthy eating style that they *want* to maintain, which makes them more likely to succeed in reaching their nutritional health goals. Now it's your turn. Let's examine what a healthy diet *really* means.

Food Guides

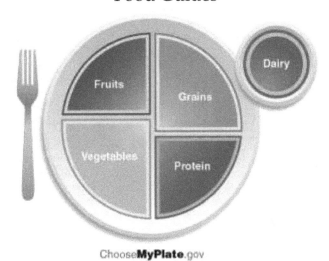

ChooseMyPlate.gov

United States Department of Agriculture (USDA) "My Plate"

The widely used U.S. government-issued Food Guide has some caveats and is an oversimplification of the complexities of nutrition, but can still be a useful guide for what to eat.

The 1995 edition of the USDA Food Guide recommended much greater amounts of bread, cereal, and pasta than the current guide, which is now referred to as "My Plate." Some argue the new guide does not adequately consider health risks associated with consuming large amounts of red and processed meat, and it still suggests consuming dairy, which is unnecessary in the diet (technically so is meat and there is more on this later in the chapter).

To address these concerns, the Harvard School of Medicine came up with its own version of "The Plate" in 2011. Both "Plates" contain useful information and illustrate important and simple concepts many people find helpful.

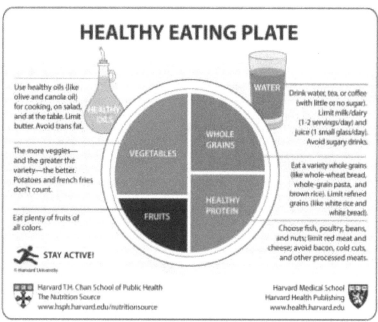

Harvard "Healthy Eating Plate"

Vegetable Category

Vegetables are the one food group most people are missing in their diets. Of the food groups, vegetables are arguably the best source of vitamins and minerals. Not consuming enough vegetables explains why many of us are sick and tired, literally. Vegetables are miraculous in all that they do for us and are delicious, but are too often considered boring and mandatory.

The number one vegetable consumed in America is... drum roll please... the french fry. Surprise!

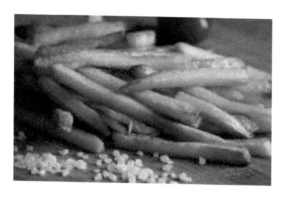

The Harvard Healthy Eating Plate doesn't count potatoes as vegetables because they break down more quickly and can affect blood sugar more dramatically than other vegetables. To this end and, for the purpose of building a balanced "Plate," potatoes should probably be considered more of a grain than a vegetable. In other words, meat and potatoes won't cut it: we also need green things on our plate.

Potatoes themselves are not bad for you. However, when potatoes are fried or processed into potato chips, nutrients are lost, fat and calories are added, and harmful substances like acrylamide (a potentially toxic and cancer-causing substance) are created.

Healthfully cooked potatoes (e.g., baked or steamed) are a good source of vitamin B6, vitamin C, potassium, copper, manganese, phosphorus, niacin, dietary fiber, and pantothenic acid.

Recommendations

One should make at least one-quarter of the total daily intake vegetables, or approximately two to three cups per day. Go for colorful varieties of whole, organic vegetables when possible. Fresh is best, frozen is OK, and canned, preferably with low sodium, is better than no vegetables.

Fruit Category

Fruits, like vegetables, are one of the most nutritious foods in existence, which is why roughly one-quarter of the "Plate" is fruit.

The Forbidden Fruit? To Eat or Not to Eat

Due to the sugar content of fruit, some argue we should eliminate this food group altogether. I disagree, unless a health condition is present that requires limiting fruit or sugar. Fruits contain vitamins, minerals, water, and fiber—nutrients most Americans are deficient in. Yes, fruit generally contains more sugar than vegetables, but the fiber in whole fruit helps the body digest the natural sugar in fruit more slowly.

Fruit Juice

Since fruit juice has had the fiber removed, it causes more of a sugar spike than whole fruit and so should be limited. Fruit juice can contain as much sugar as soda—but it does contain more vitamins and minerals; so, between the two, juice is a healthier choice.

Beth's Healthy Spritzer (page 48) is a great way to limit sugary fruit juice and get some of the important vitamins and minerals that come from fruit.

Recommendations

Go for whole, organic whenever possible, fruits and strive to "eat the rainbow," as different colored foods contain different nutrients. It is generally recommended to consume one and one half to two cups of fruit per day, or one-quarter of total intake.

Grain Category

No more than one-quarter of our "plate" or daily intake should be grains, and only half of that (one-eighth) should be refined or processed grains. Should we call the grain police on you? Luckily, there are no such police, or many of us would be locked up in food jail. Although, I would argue that many of our bodies are incarcerated in the prison of *imbalance*.

Whole (ideally organic), diversified grains in moderation can be an important building block of an overall healthy diet. However, most Americans eat too many grains, especially refined grains. We should choose mostly whole grains and expand the varieties, such as amaranth, barley, brown rice, millet, oats, quinoa, and others. Overly processed, overly consumed, nutrient-deficient grains (like white flour and white rice) should be limited. There is more on processed grains in the next chapter.

Lectins: What Are They and Are They Bad for Me?

Lectins, a type of protein found in many foods, but especially prominent in grains and beans, are being "blamed" for a variety of health problems: from digestive distress and skin irritations to brain fog, chronic fatigue, and inflammation. Many health experts, including me, believe all of the fuss over lectins is overblown.

First, cooking vastly reduces the lectin content of many foods. Second, lectins may have health benefits. Lectins that are found in legumes have antimicrobial features and act as anti-cancer agents. Additionally, beans, peas, and lentils have been shown to reduce blood pressure and inflammation. As they are high in fiber and have a low glycemic index, these foods can also be helpful in regulating blood sugar levels.

Someone with a chronic digestion problem (e.g., irritable bowel syndrome) or an autoimmune condition (e.g., rheumatoid arthritis) might consider an elimination diet or talking to their healthcare provider about the possibility of removing lectin-rich foods from their diet. However, although some people may be sensitive to lectins, that does not mean that they are toxic or that most people should avoid them.

The bottom line is that food sensitivities, including to grains and ingredients within them such as lectins, usually have more to do with overconsumption of adulterated food and compromised immunity due to consuming these foods than with any one ingredient, food type or food group.[1]

Recommendations

Again, the recommended amount for grains is no more than one-quarter of total daily intake. In terms of ounces that is six ounces per day for a 2,000 calorie per day diet. One ounce is about one small six-inch tortilla or one slice of bread about the size of a cassette tape. As mentioned previously, most Americans exceed those recommended amounts by far, especially with regard to *processed* grains.

Protein Category

Protein was also discussed in Macronutrients chapter. Again, protein is an important nutrient, but most Americans eat too much, and from unhealthy sources such as bacon, sausage, cold cuts, other processed meats, and excess amounts of red meat. There are many plant-based options as well as healthier animal sources of protein.

The fact that most Americans get the bulk of their protein from animals can be problematic for several reasons, including how the animals are *raised* and *processed*.

Conventionally raised animals are often raised in unhealthy, toxic, and even inhumane ways. Ideally, animal food products: eggs, meat, and dairy, should come from healthy, ethically, and sustainably raised animals that are fed healthy and appropriate foods; are antibiotic, steroid, pesticide, insecticide, and GMO free; and are consumed in balance with the other food groups.

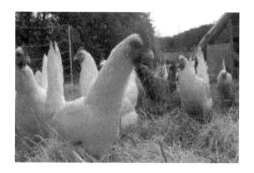

Healthier Edible Animals

The USDA's definition of "Free Range" or "Free Roaming" chicken is that "the poultry has been allowed access to the outside."

"Providing access to the outside" could mean that there is a small door somewhere in the shed. It does not mean that the birds ever exit the shed. "Outside" could mean a small concrete slab. Therefore, the term "free range" is often meaningless. "Pasture-raised" is more likely to mean access to pasture, which is much healthier for the animal.[2,3]

One website dedicated to healthy raising practices says animals should graze on "grassy pastures where they hunt, peck, scratch, and eat grasses, weeds, flowers, bugs, grubs, and anything else out there that piques their fancy."[4]

Healthy poultry is not raised in an artificial, chemically-laden, crowded, and overly-controlled environment.

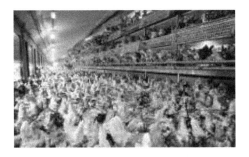

Efficiency is an important aspect of any business; however there should be ethical limits. Raising healthier animals will benefit the physical and mental health of the animals, humans who eat them, farm workers, as well as the farms and the planet.

Recommendations

Approximately one-quarter of the plate or total daily intake should be composed of healthy protein sources. There are more detailed recommendations for Protein in the Macronutrients chapter.

Dairy/Water Category

The term "dairy" includes milk and any food products, such as cheese, cream, butter, and yogurt; produced from the milk of mammals such as cows and goats.

As I have mentioned, humans do not need to consume animal products, including dairy, to survive. Health and ethical issues such as should we really be drinking the breast milk of another animal meant for her baby, could be solved by eliminating milk products from our diets.

If we don't need to consume dairy why does the USDA Food Guide include it? The answer is that the glass of milk on the "My Plate" was largely a result of "lobbying" by the dairy industry, and probably some nutritional ignorance on the part of the decision makers.

The main reasons milk is recommended are the protein and calcium content of dairy products. However, there is as much calcium in a half cup of tofu as there is in one cup of milk. Bok choy, kale, turnip greens, chickpeas, and salmon are also great sources of calcium. We can get sufficient protein from plants sources. Additionally, milk contains sugar (lactose) and simple carbs which we should limit. A better name for this category would be "Healthy Beverages."

Drinking healthy beverages including water, tea, and plant-based milks such as almond, coconut, hemp, or rice is healthier and cheaper. Unopened containers can last for weeks or months. Furthermore, no animal had to lactate to produce them. Skip sugary drinks, limit juice to a small glass per day, and, if you do consume animal milk products, make them organic whenever possible and limit them to no more than one to two servings a day.

Oils

The Harvard "Plate" lists various oils and says we "should not be afraid to cook with vegetable oils." However, we do not actually *need* oil. Healthy fats come from whole foods including avocados, olives, nuts, and seeds.

The Hype about Coconut Oil

Coconut oil is one of the rare plant foods that contain saturated fat and, as mentioned earlier, consuming limited amounts of saturated fat is considered to be fine by most nutrition experts.

The chemical bonds in unsaturated fats are less stable than in saturated fats, so they break apart more easily. Broken bonds can lead to the formation of free radicals which are thought to lead to health issues such as inflammation, dementia, and premature aging. However, these weaker bonds are also part of what makes unsaturated fats so healthy *and* help combat those same illnesses.

Another reason for the hype is that some people are touting saturated fat as the "new miracle nutrient," which is unproven. The bottom line is this: unless you are frying food regularly, which is not healthy anyway, you probably do not need to be concerned about the heat tolerances of chemical bonds in fats.

To eliminate the confusion and need for oil altogether, try coating with a healthy oil and baking or sautéing food in vegetable broth. If you do use oil, I recommend quality oils such as extra virgin olive oil for cooking at low temperatures and cold foods, and avocado or coconut oils for cooking at high temperatures. There is more detail on oils in the "Fats" section of the Macronutrients chapter.

Plate Size Matters

The overall surface area of an average American dinner plate has increased almost 40 percent since 1960. Plate sizes have grown from nine to 12 inches in homes and now average 13 inches in restaurants. The 1960 portions would look minuscule on today's larger plates.

Research shows that people are inclined to eat more food if more is on their plate. More food satisfies both eyes and stomach, and the brain learns it takes more food to be satisfying.[5]

We often hear terms such as "jumbo," "ultimate," "colossal," and "all you can eat." Since the 1970's, as a result of all of this "supersizing," Americans' daily caloric intake has gone from 2,200 to 2,700 per person.[6]

Here are some examples of serving size increases:

Food	1970 calories	2016 calories
Cheeseburger	300	600
French fries	200	600
Muffin	200	500
Pasta plate	500	1000
Soda	85	250
Theater popcorn	300	600
Turkey sandwich	300	800

In addition to the growing serving sizes, much of the food in the "Western" diet is less nutritious than it once was. Necessary nutrients like fiber, vitamins, minerals, and amino acids are removed from most foods and sugar, fat, salt, and other substances are added. The body then craves more as it seeks to nourish itself and the taste buds want more of the tantalizing, maniacally contrived concoctions—and it has worked: people are eating more than ever!

This "junk" food fantasy is leading to obesity, diabetes, high cholesterol, and other health problems. However, at least the fast-food giants and food manufacturers are doing well!

The "Plates" Can Provide Much Needed Clarity

There is a lot of confusion about nutrition today and many people are in desperate need of clarity. The "Plates," though imperfect, used intelligently and as guides, can help. We could solve many of our health problems just by following these guides more closely. For example, to eat about half of our daily intake of fruits and vegetables and no more than one-eighth of our daily intake in the form of processed grains would be a big improvement for most people.

The next time you see a popular American fast food ad, compare it to the "Plate" guides, and see which food groups are missing and which are overrepresented. I have visions of pepperoni pizza, pasta, cheesy bread sticks, chicken wings, fried chicken, biscuits, cookies, cake, and soda dancing in my head. You?

Popular Diets—Sorting through the Noise

I am often asked about diets such as high carb, low carb, high protein, high fat, and gluten-free. My advice is almost always the same: balance. Many people are eating too much of certain types of foods and not enough of the foods with nutrients our bodies need to function. Therefore, and as I have said, many people's diets are out of balance.

Though many diet books make good points, they often focus on just one nutrient, food, or problem. The proposed solutions in the vast majority of diet books out there are trying to address these imbalances, but they often only add to the confusion.

The pendulum of imbalance continues to swing back and forth, from low-fat to high-fat and all the other diet fads in between. The true way forward is knowledge and, I'll say it again (and again), *balance.*

The answer to the vacuum of missing information is access to honest, accurate nutrition information.

Making the Grade—Ranking Popular Diets

U.S. News and World Report looked at 40 popular diets and had them graded by a panel of nationally recognized experts in diet, nutrition, obesity, food psychology, diabetes, and heart disease. The experts looked at nutritional completeness, health risks, long and short term results, and how easy a diet is to follow, among other criteria.[7]

The good news is that all the top ranking diets involved a balanced, healthy approach to food and included healthy options from the food groups. Here are the winners and some highlights from the report.

#1 *The Mediterranean Diet (tied for first)*

The Mediterranean Diet, which features meals high in "good" fats, ranked as the top diet on the *U.S. News and World Report's* ranking. This popular diet tied with The DASH Diet for first place. The Mediterranean Diet recommends emulating how people in the Mediterranean region have traditionally eaten, with a focus on foods such as olive oil, fish, and vegetables. The report called the diet a "well-balanced eating plan."

#1 *The DASH Diet (tied for first)*

The DASH Diet has been ranked as the top overall diet by the Report for eight consecutive rankings. Originating from the National Heart, Lung, and Blood Institute (NHLBI) as a way to help reduce blood pressure, the DASH Diet is based on low-sodium and healthful foods. It recommends fruit, vegetables, whole grains, lean protein, and low-fat dairy, and eliminates foods and drinks high in fat, sugar, and salt.

#3: *The Flexitarian Diet*

The Flexitarian Diet encourages people to try alternative meat options such as tofu but leaves room for flexibility if you can't quite fully give up meat. The diet allows you to reap the benefits of a plant-heavy diet and still eat meat occasionally. This plant-heavy diet focuses on adding foods to your diet such as the "new meats" (tofu, beans, lentils, peas, nuts and seeds, and eggs), fruits and vegetables, whole grains, dairy, and sugar and spices — instead of taking foods away.

Weight Watchers (in the top five)

Weight Watchers ranked in the top five for best diets overall and also obtained the number one ranking for best commercial diet and best fast weight-loss diet this year. The program focuses on assigning points based on the nutritional value of foods. The points are greater for foods high in saturated fats and sugars, and lower for foods with high levels of protein. The downsides of this diet are that it requires a membership fee and once the program is suspended the weight returns for many dieters.

In Last Place: The Keto and Whole 30 Diets

One of the concerns about the Keto Diet is that it is high in saturated fat. Generally, Keto Diets recommend that 60 to 75 percent of calories come from fat which is contrary to the American Heart Association's recommended 20 to 35 percent. Experts say the diet can be especially dangerous for people with or those prone to develop, severe diabetes, kidney disease, and heart disease.

The Whole30 Diet, which gets 60,000 searches per month on Google, eliminates food groups including sugar, grains, dairy and legumes for 30 days; hence the name "Whole30."

The expert panel of nutritionists, dietary consultants, and physicians assessing each of these diets says the Keto and Whole30 are both "fad diets" that unnecessarily wipe out entire food groups, and that is not safe or healthy.[7,8]

Other Popular Concepts

Calorie Counting

A calorie is an accurate form of energy measurement, but it is virtually useless as a form of nutrient measurement. Many dietitians say, "A calorie is a calorie," which implies that all you need to concern yourself with in your diet is the number of calories you consume. This is a simple approach for those concerned with losing weight, but it is not enough.

The calorie-counting approach is simple — too simple — and that is why calorie counting alone to lose weight often doesn't work.

For instance, many people avoid fat because it is high in calories. Fat *does* contain more calories than carbohydrates or protein, but it is also very satisfying. It's denser, so we require less of it in order to feel full. Plus, we *need* fat, just in the right amounts.

When I received my nutrition education, no one said to me, "A calorie is a calorie. Now go count the calories for all your patients." If all that mattered were calories, I would have been better off with a math degree, not a pre-med degree.

A lack of true nutrition knowledge in our society, combined with our short attention span, has created a need for brief, convenient answers — hence, the calorie counting obsession. If calorie counting was all we needed to be concerned about, we could just eat doughnuts, hot dogs, and other unhealthy foods all the time as long as we stayed within the calorie limit. For example, a friend who was on a calorie or "point-based" diet would skip meals and drink her "points" in beer.

The goal is to get the proper amount of nutrients, not just the proper amount of calories.

The theory behind calorie counting is that successful calorie counters will consume more nutritious foods such as fruits and vegetables which generally have fewer calories than unhealthy foods. This is a good theory, but it only works if people understand these principles and how to apply them.

To Cleanse or Not to Cleanse

As incidences of health problems such as leaky gut, colitis, irritable bowel syndrome, depression, anxiety, autoimmune disorders, fatigue, and food allergies become more prevalent, people often look to dietary "cleanses" as a solution.

Many health issues today *are* related to poor diet, so a healthy, safe, evidence-based detox program to cleanse the body makes sense for some people. However, the best way to stay "clean" is to limit processed and other "toxic" foods and eat plenty of whole plant foods which have built-in detoxification mechanisms including vitamins, minerals, fiber, and water.

Weight-Loss Cleanses

Drastic "weight loss" cleanses are definitely not a good idea. Rapid weight loss is unsustainable *and* unhealthy, as it results in mostly water and muscle loss. Our bodies need water to function and for weight loss, and muscle helps burn fat, so losing water and muscle is *not* helpful for long-term weight loss.

Healthy, long-term fat weight loss is gradual, typically only about one to two pounds a week. Healthy weight loss occurs naturally by adhering to a healthy lifestyle and by giving the body the nutrition it needs.

Some cleanses may give instant apparent results but are dangerous and are likely to sabotage any future weight loss efforts. Starvation diets and cleanses simply "mess" with the metabolism and the body's ability to burn calories. Extreme diets teach the body to hang onto excess calories as reserves in case it is ever "starved" again. Or as I tell my students, similar to how a chipmunk stores food for winter.

Fasting

Fasting is done for health and religious reasons. It is often done as a form of cleanse. Advocates claim fasting can effectively treat many medical conditions, including arthritis, depression, digestive disorders, eczema, heart disease, and high blood pressure.[9]

A periodic, healthy fast or "cleanse" can give the organs a rest, reboot the system, and purge unwanted toxins.

I did a healthy fast myself years ago because I felt I needed it, and I felt it was beneficial. Now, I try to consistently keep my body "clean" by consuming a whole, unadulterated, mostly plant food diet and trying to drink plenty of quality water. I may do another cleanse soon to give my organs a rest from processing solid foods, but I will also give my body lots of liquid nutrients throughout the entire cleanse as I did the last time. That, along with your own intuition, is what I recommend for anyone considering a healthy, periodic fast.

Plant-Based Diets

All of the nutrients our bodies need can be found in non-animal sources. Vegan, vegetarian, and plant-based diets have been proven to be highly effective for weight loss, and plant-based eaters have lower rates of diabetes, heart disease, and obesity.[10]

Those who eat only plant-sourced foods are called "plant-based" or "vegan eaters." However, the term "vegan" refers to someone who does not consume or *use* any animal or animal tested products. "Vegetarians" eat some animal products such as eggs, milk, and cheese. There are also "pescatarians" who consume fish as their only meat source and "lacto/ovo vegetarians" who consume milk and eggs, but no meat. "Omnivores" consume animal as well as vegetable products.

It is, of course, possible to eat an unhealthy "plant" diet. After all, a diet consisting of soda pop and chips is vegan![2] Healthy, plant-based diets include plenty of nutrient-dense plant foods including vegetables, whole grains, fruits, and legumes, and minimal oils, processed foods, and animal foods including meat, eggs and dairy products.[10]

Personally, I consume about a 90 percent plant-based diet. Learning to buy and cook with only plants has been a fun, satisfying, sometimes frustrating, ultimately liberating adventure. A healthy plant-based diet generally includes more fiber, vitamins and minerals, and healthy essential fats than a typical animal-based diet. Plant-based diets can also save time, money, and hassle.

For instance, plant-based products are generally less expensive than animal-based products. There is less worry about cross-contamination and cooking food sufficiently to destroy the bacteria found in animal products. This reduces meal preparation and cooking time and eliminates the extra effort, worry, *and* health risks associated with food-borne illnesses.

I am continually learning, evolving, and striving to keep things in balance, which means I occasionally eat animal products, and I think of it as a treat.

I don't preach to others to become entirely "vegan" eaters and most experts agree that eating meat and other animal products in moderation is fine. However, I do preach that most people should eat more whole plant products because most are lacking in that area. For those that consume animal products, I recommend choosing products made from the healthiest and most ethically raised and processed animals, as mentioned earlier.

Many "vegan" meal and recipe ideas can be found in Appendix A.

Clean Eating

The term "clean eating" has gained in popularity recently. "Clean eating" is the same as what I and many other nutritionists advocate: to eat more natural, healthy, whole foods including vegetables, fruits, and whole grains; incorporate healthy proteins and fat; and cut back on refined grains, additives, preservatives, unhealthy fats, and large amounts of added sugar and salt.[11] These are the "nuts and bolts" of good nutrition.

Why Diets Don't Work: What Does Work

A desire for drastic change and fast results explain the popularity of many diets. However, many of these diets are not only unhealthy but they don't work long-term because they focus on surface changes based on minimal information, and *avoiding* many foods.

Most diets involve deprivation and will power, so weight loss is usually temporary. Dieters are often sold pre-packaged food and given specific instructions, and told what foods to eat and to avoid, and the weight usually returns once the program is discontinued.

The key to long-term weight management is through sustainable lifestyle changes that come from understanding what, when, why, and how to eat.

Thinking about food from a positive standpoint, and focusing on what to eat, instead of what *not* to eat, creates options, not restrictions. And after learning how to eat healthy based on a nutrition *education*, one usually *wants* to because an optimally functioning body feels good.

I work with my clients to customize diet plans based on *their* lifestyle and preferences. They learn how to eat healthy in a comfortable way. The goal is that they will ultimately "graduate" and be equipped to "do it themselves" economically and long term. This "education" includes customized meal plans we create together, and clear nutrition information, which makes the client much more likely to reach and sustain their health goals, all without a lifetime membership fee.

However, proper nutrition education and personal nutrition counseling are not financial options for many people today, and this should change. I advocate for this throughout this book and my career.

Creative Meal Planning: My 80/20 Formula

Okay, okay, so, what *should* you eat?!

After years of intensive study, I devised a simple plan for healthy eating which I called the 80/20 formula. The 80/20 method is popular because it includes simple rules one can follow without being deprived of their favorite foods.

One can eat more than just plain carrots, salad, celery sticks, baked skinless chicken breast, and meal replacement shakes in order to "eat healthy" *or* "lose weight," although that may be what one expects to hear from a *dietitian*.

The 80/20 formula means bending the rules 20 percent of the time and doing what is right for the rest. For example, one soda per day would be close to consuming 20 percent of the daily limit for "bad" foods, and much of the rest of the day would need to be spent eating nutritiously. However, what does *nutritiously* mean?

Most of us are not getting the nutrients our bodies need. For many, a standard fast food meal is a burger, fries, and soda—which is roughly

1,400 calories at McDonald's.[12] Assuming they had a daily caloric requirement of 2,000 calories (the midpoint of 1,600 to 2,400, which is what most adults need), eating just two of these meals a day already puts them over the daily limit by 800 calories. This meal is also high in saturated fat, sugar, salt, and cholesterol—all the "bad" stuff that can lead to conditions such as obesity, diabetes, and hypertension.

It is theoretically possible to consume a fast food meal—or any other "unhealthy" meal—as part of the 80/20 program. However, these foods are so high in calories they do not leave room for much else and they often create cravings for more. So, eating them can sabotage the will to stick to *any* program. However, the fact is that balance can be found and deprivation can be alleviated in many instances.

The truth is that *eating* food can lead to better health and a healthy weight, but it depends on what, how much, and when. The 80/20 formula allows for flexibility to consume foods we love. Unfortunately, many people have the 80/20 in reverse and don't know it or understand how to achieve a healthy balance in a satisfying way.

Healthy eating means consuming a variety of minimally processed or "whole" foods with healthy representations from each of the food groups (protein, grains, fruits, and vegetables) in a balanced way at least 80 percent of the time.

Focus on What We Can Eat

Make a plan to fill in the 80 percent with foods you enjoy, and then have fun—enjoying the freedom and spontaneity that comes with the rest. So, when you are unexpectedly offered dessert at a party, you can say, "Yes!" without overthinking or worrying it because you know you have been mostly "good."

Eat as many healthy, whole plant foods as desired, unless there is a health condition or other reason to limit certain foods. Plant foods help nourish the body and create the feeling of satiety (satisfaction) because these foods contain many nutrients our bodies know they need.

We must be realistic to succeed. An 80/20 (or 90/10 for the high achievers, as long as it is sustainable) ratio plan is much more realistic than trying not to eat butter, chocolate, ice cream, or whatever your favorite food is, ever again.

100/0

I do *not* advocating eating food with chemical additives. The ultimate goal when it comes to consuming "strange substances" in our food should be absolutely zero or "100/0." However, as will be discussed in upcoming chapters, making our food supply 100 percent "strange substance" free will require focus. Until this happens, we should all do our best to limit these unhealthy ingredients from our diets altogether. In other words, try to make the bacon, wine, or chocolate cake organic!

Finding a Fun Balance

A balanced diet can still contain things we like, and lots of people like pizza. Many are surprised to learn they can still eat pizza as part of a healthy diet.

In fact, there are many "tricks" of the nutrition trade that help make healthy eating sustainable. Here are some ways to include pizza in a healthy diet:

#1: choose whole-grain and/or thin crust
#2: load up on vegetables
#3: choose lean instead of fatty meats
#4: add a side salad — dipped (not drenched) in your favorite dressing

There are many more tricks and they all relate to keeping a healthy balance.

- Diversify ingredients, foods, and food groups.
- Eat breakfast! A small, healthy meal in the morning turns on the metabolism for the day.
- Eat at least three, up to six, small meals throughout the day rather

than one or two large ones. This helps keep the metabolism turned on which helps the body burn fat, and supports the multitude of body processes happening all the time.

- Find what works for you!

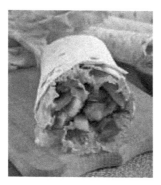

A Balanced Wrap (try chicken or plant-based meat)

Here is a sample two-day menu following the 80/20 plan.

Plant-based or other substitutions based on personal preferences can be made (which is the whole point of the 80/20 plan). This menu is based on how I ate when I consumed more animal products than I do now. This menu is more representative of the amount of animal foods most people choose to eat today, so it is a good starting point. There are also several plant-based meal ideas listed in Appendix A.

Day One

Breakfast
1 cup whole-grain cereal or oatmeal with honey* to taste
1/2 peach or other fruit
1-2 cups water, *Beth's Healthy Spritzer* (page 48), coffee or tea

Snack
3/4 cup cottage cheese with fruit (try pineapple; or avocado, tomato, and green onions with a pinch of salt and pepper)

Lunch

1 tuna salad sandwich on whole-grain bread with tomatoes, lettuce and 2 tsp. of regular mayonnaise* or plain yogurt
1 serving Sunchips, baked or regular chips*
1 cup water, herbal tea, or *Beth's Healthy Spritzer*
1 apple, orange, or other fruit

Snack

1-2 stalks celery with cream cheese* or peanut butter or 8-10 baby carrot sticks w/ranch dressing*

Dinner

1 chicken breast sautéed in olive or canola oil and fresh herbs such as oregano or rosemary
1 cup roasted red potatoes with olive or canola oil, pepper, and salt*
1 cup sautéed or baked asparagus with olive oil and lemon pepper

Dessert

3/4 cup ice cream* or 1-2 cookies*

Day Two

Breakfast

1 egg*
1 piece of whole-grain toast with canola oil margarine
1 banana
1 cup coffee, tea, or *Beth's Healthy Spritzer*

Snack

1/2 cup plain or vanilla* yogurt with fresh or frozen blueberries and maple syrup* or honey* to taste (for plain yogurt)

Lunch

1 cup whole-grain pasta with marinara sauce or 2 slices pizza*
1 cup romaine lettuce, Caesar salad dressing*, croutons*, parmesan cheese
1-2 cups water flavored with lemon or *Beth's Healthy Spritzer*

Snack

3/4 cup almonds and dried cranberries or other trail mix

Dinner
1 eggplant or steak* with lobster tail* or shrimp* with vegetables and potato or brown or white* rice
1-2 pieces of white* or whole-wheat bread with olive oil, butter*, or margarine*
1-2 drinks of choice (water, juice*, soda*, milk*, wine*, beer*, or *Beth's Healthy Spritzer*)
Dessert
3/4 cup frozen yogurt* or other low-fat dessert*

Note: Serving sizes vary depending on gender, age, weight, etc. Items with an asterisk (*) are in the "bad" or 20 percent column for various reasons, such as sugar, saturated or trans-fat, cholesterol, salt, white flour or preservative content.

"Day Two" has the option for steak, lobster or shrimp, eggs, and butter. These foods are all high in cholesterol. Because this menu includes these foods, the next day would not be a good day for more high-cholesterol foods. Instead, lean protein sources and lots of fruits and vegetables would be great choices.

Stay Active for Healthy Weight Maintenance

Exercise is extremely important for health and weight maintenance. Research has shown that, for weight loss to be permanent, it must be followed up with sufficient cardiovascular exercise to maintain it. Basically, fat cells are hardy little buggers and they *want* to survive. The data shows that sufficient exercise to sustain weight loss equates to 150 minutes of moderate-intensity aerobic activity, 75 minutes of vigorous-intensity aerobic activity, or an equivalent mix of the two, per week.[13] The lack of consistent and sufficient exercise is probably one reason many people do not achieve and maintain weight loss.

So Much Passion!

There are many passionately-held dietary beliefs, such as vegan, vegetarian, omnivore, high fat, high protein, low carb, anti-grain, no-sugar, and so on. This book is intended to share the nuts and bolts of nutrition, and again, not go into depth about *every* nutritional issue or diet fad.

Important concepts are covered here to provide a foundation from which decisions about what to eat can be made based on personal preferences and knowledge, not on hype, hysteria, or emotion.

A nutrition *education,* where one learns about healthy eating and then can make sustainable lifestyle changes, is far superior to yo-yo dieting or trying each new "quick fix" diet fad, hoping the next one will be "the one."

There is more information on healthy eating, including recipes and articles, on my website (Anutritionrevolution.com) and in Appendix A.

Chapter Seven

Processed Food:
Nutritional Mayhem

"The food you eat can either be the safest and most powerful form of medicine, or the slowest form of poison."
– Ann Wigmore

Processed food is defined as raw food that has been adulterated or modified to increase its nutritional content or make it more palatable and easier to ship and sell. Scientists are still learning about the many nutrients in foods, so we often don't even know what we are "processing" out of our foods.

Food is heated for taste and texture and to kill dangerous pathogens. However, heat also destroys *nutrients* because the bonds that hold the nutrients together are broken and they die. Cooking can cause a nutrient loss of up to 80 percent in vegetables. Heat can be good, but what is being destroyed *along* with the pathogens should also give us concern.

Food manufacturers work hard to make their food *addictive*. A phrase on a popular potato chip commercial says, "You can't eat just one." This is not an accident.

As a result of consuming large amounts of highly processed foods, many Americans are now overfed and undernourished. Research has shown that there is a 14 percent risk of early death with every 10 percent increase in consumption of ultra-processed foods.[1]

Whole, raw food is naturally rich in many nutrients. Those nutrients give the body what it needs to function and less of the substances that make it sick.

Our bodies understand whole foods. Whole foods don't confuse the system like overly manipulated processed foods do. Whole foods heal and satisfy us and give us what we need. They don't trick us or unnaturally addict us.

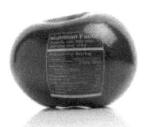

Let's look at some examples. First, here is a list to compare the nutrients lost by processing whole apples into sauce and juice.

Nutrient	Units	Whole Apple	Applesauce	Apple Juice
Macronutrient				
Fiber	G	3	2	0
Sugars	G	14	23	13
Minerals				
Beta Carotene	Mcg	37	0	0
Choline	Mg	5	0	3
Fluoride	Mcg	5	0	0
Folate	Mcg	4	1	0
Lutein	Mcg	40	0	22
Magnesium	Mg	7	4	7
Phosphorus	Mg	15	10	10
Potassium	Mg	148	84	139
Sodium	Mg	1	39	6
Vitamin A	IU	75	15	1
	RAE, Mcg	4	1	0
Vitamin C	Mg	6	2	1
Vitamin K	Mcg	3	0	0

Note: Amounts are based on a medium apple (138 grams).[2]

Refined Wheat Grain, A.K.A. "White" Flour

White flour is used to make most bread products on the market today. It is being processed in a way that makes it unhealthy *and* addicting.

White flour contains less fiber and protein and other nutrients that help us feel satisfied. We reach for more and actually *crave* more, and of course, the product manufacturers make more money.

Wheat is being subsidized by the government which has led to more wheat on the market today than most other grains. There is more on this later.

As illustrated in the Amino Acid chapter, white flour contains one part of the grain, the endosperm, which is the part with the least nutritional value.

Let's investigate by comparing the nutritional differences between whole-wheat flour and refined or "white" flour.

Nutrient	Units	Whole-Wheat Flour	White Flour
Macronutrients			
Energy	kCal	407	455
Protein	G	16.44	12.91
Carbohydrate	G	87.08	95.39
Fiber	G	14.6	3.4
Minerals			
Calcium	Mg	41	19
Iron	Mg	4.66	1.46
Magnesium	Mg	166	28
Phosphorus	Mg	415	135
Potassium	Mg	486	134
Sodium	Mg	6	2
Zinc	Mg	3.52	0.88
Copper	Mg	0.458	0.180

Manganese	Mg	4.559	0.853
Selenium	Mcg	84.8	42.4
Vitamins			
Thiamin	Mg	0.536	0.150
Riboflavin	Mg	0.258	0.050
Niacin	Mg	7.638	1.562
Pantothenic acid	Mg	1.210	0.547
Vitamin B-6	Mg	0.409	0.055
Folate	Mcg	53	32
Choline	Mg	37.4	13.0
Betaine	Mg	87.4	0.0
Carotene, beta	Mcg	6	0
Vitamin A	IU	11	0
Lutein + zeaxanthin	Mcg	264	22
Vitamin E (alpha-tocopherol)	Mg	0.98	0.07
Vitamin K (phylloquinone)	Mcg	2.3	0.4
Fats			
Fatty acids, saturated	G	0.386	0.194
Fatty acids, mono-unsaturated	G	0.278	0.109
Fatty acids, poly-unsaturated	G	0.935	0.516
Amino acids			
Tryptophan	G	0.254	0.159
Threonine	G	0.474	0.351
Isoleucine	G	0.610	0.446
Leucine	G	1.111	0.887
Lysine	G	0.454	0.285
Methionine	G	0.254	0.229
Cystine	G	0.380	0.274

Phenylalanine	G	0.775	0.650
Tyrosine	G	0.480	0.390
Valine	G	0.742	0.519
Arginine	G	0.770	0.521
Histidine	G	0.380	0.287
Alanine	G	0.584	0.415
Aspartic acid	G	0.844	0.544
Glutamic acid	G	5.190	4.349
Glycine	G	0.662	0.464
Proline	G	1.706	1.498
Serine	G	0.775	0.645

Note: Amounts are based on a one-cup serving.[2]

As evidenced by this list, whole-wheat flour has many more nutrients than its overly processed counterpart, making it far more nutritious. Wheat also contains gluten, as discussed earlier in the Amino Acids chapter. Many people are developing intolerances to gluten as a result of overproducing, overmanipulating, and overconsuming white flour. Adding to the problem, most conventionally grown wheat is grown with toxic chemicals including pesticides.

Did you notice that this list is much longer than on standard food labels? Our bodies need and crave all these nutrients, not just a few, so we should consider and consume them *all*. We should also consider what in the heck we are doing to our food.

Strange Substances in Food Supply

Our nutritional problems often relate to adulterated food. Man and all of our machines have made many advancements, for better *and* worse. A manufacturing revolution has brought much progress and efficiency, but has also destroyed the nutritional integrity and health of numerous plants, animals, humans, and parts of the planet.

Pesticides in produce, hormones in milk, and antibiotics in meat are just some of the adulterations occurring in food production today. Research on the effects of all this manipulation is limited, and most studies done on the safety of these foreign substances are supported by the food manufacturing companies themselves.[3]

Much of the conventionally produced food is unhealthy and unsafe. More than 10,000 substances qualify as allowable additives to food. However, these substances have been linked to various health problems. Many other health problems from the effects of these substances, their cumulative effect, and effect in conjunction with each other are no doubt yet to be discovered.[4]

Some additives are used to increase shelf life, improve taste, imitate natural flavors, and make money. Here is a glimpse into some of the unnatural substances in our food supply:

Antibiotics

Livestock producers routinely give antibiotics to animals so they grow faster and to keep them from developing illnesses from crowded, stressful, and unsanitary conditions.[5]

The overuse of antibiotics is creating "superbugs" which are deadly bacteria that are resistant to the antibiotics. The World Health Organization (WHO) says antibiotic resistance is "one of the biggest threats to global health, food security, and development today," and leads to longer hospital stays, higher medical costs, and more deaths from antibiotic resistant infections.

Despite this, the U.S. government has not yet issued enforceable regulations on antibiotics in food animals. Instead, they publish "voluntary guidelines."[6] Companies aren't obligated to label their meat or provide information regarding their use of antibiotics to consumers.

Artificial Colors

The purpose of artificial colors is to mimic natural ones. Synthetic colors have been implicated in negative effects on children's behavior including hyperactivity, and combinations of artificial colors and other additives have been found to cause tumors.[4]

GMOs

What is a GMO? Genetically Modified (or engineered) Organisms ("GM" or "GMO") are defined as those in which the genetic material ("DNA") has been altered in such a way that does not occur naturally. The goals of GM foods are improved nutrition and taste, decreased reliance on pesticides, increased tolerance to drought, increased yield, and decreased production costs.

Modifying the genetic material of living things comes with risks. Some of the risks of GM foods include unwanted changes in nutritional content, the creation of allergens, and toxic effects on bodily organs, less resistance of crops to certain pests, and cross-pollinating with traditional crops, which could potentially lead to the extinction of some organisms, as well as other unexpected outcomes.[7]

The New York Times reports that "90 percent of scientists believe GMOs are safe." However, according to the same article, two-thirds of the public does not agree.[8]

Evidence is still being collected, and more research and time are needed to fully understand the implications of GMOs.

High Fructose Corn Syrup (HFCS)

High fructose corn syrup is a substance made from corn starch with enzymes added to it to convert some of the sucrose into fructose. HFCS is structurally similar, though not identical, to table sugar (sucrose).[9]

Research shows that the sugars found in HFCS were more toxic to mice than sucrose. When scientists fed mice a human-sized dose of either sugar, they observed that the HFCS-type sugar reduced both the reproductive capacity and lifespan of female mice. Female mice fed fructose-glucose died at almost two times the rate of females on the sucrose diet. Also, mice who consumed HFCS produced 26 percent fewer offspring than those fed table sugar.[10]

Most U.S. corn, from which HFCS is derived, is GMO, so there's also *that*. There is more on HFCS in the Government chapter.

Hormones

Hormones — typically synthetic estrogens and testosterone — have been used for decades in the meat and dairy industries to increase the size of the animal and the amount of milk that dairy cows produce.
Industry-funded research shows no health risks, but independent research studies differ. Results have shown links to breast cancer, and added hormones are suspected to contribute to early puberty in children.

More research is needed, but there is already enough concern that many countries have banned the use of added hormones. No major studies are underway in the U.S. to evaluate the safety of hormones in meat and milk.[3]

Monosodium Glutamate (MSG)

In the 1960s, some people developed symptoms such as tingling, numbness, brain fog, chest pressure, and pain after eating Chinese food. This was referred to as the "Chinese Restaurant Syndrome." It was later discovered that monosodium glutamate or MSG, a common food additive, was to blame.

Research done in the 1970s, showed that MSG killed brain cells. Since the public became aware of the dangers of MSG, the names including anything hydrolyzed, sodium caseinate, and whey protein isolate have changed. So, now, it is more difficult to identify foods made with MSG. MSG is still permissible in foods as long as it is present in less than 99 percent pure amounts.[11] Again, we are not sure of the cumulative effects of the overall dietary intake of all of these compounds.

Nitrates and Other "Strange Substances" in Processed Meats

There is no clear definition for "processed meat," but anything smoked, salted, cured, or containing preservatives is processed. Bacon, hot dogs, beef jerky, chicken nuggets, pepperoni, fast food hamburgers, and lunch meats are considered "processed meats." People who eat a lot of processed meats are at increased risk of developing heart disease, diabetes, and cancer.[12]

In 2018, the World Health Organization classified processed meats as a "group one carcinogen," meaning they can cause cancer in humans.[13] Many experts, Including the American Academy of Pediatrics, recommend avoiding processed meats altogether, especially for those who are pregnant or breastfeeding.[14]

Nitrates are used for coloring, flavor, and preservation in cured meats. Nitrates help meats retain that fresh-looking pink color, even after weeks on the store shelf.

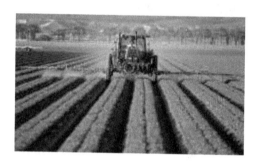

Pesticides

Pesticides are chemicals that are used to kill fungus, bacteria, insects, plant diseases, snails, slugs, or weeds, among others. These chemicals can work by ingestion or by touch and death may occur immediately or over a period of time. Insecticides are a type of pesticide that is used to specifically target and kill insects. Some insecticides include snail bait, ant killer, and wasp killer.

Herbicides are used to kill undesirable plants or "weeds." Some herbicides will kill all the plants they touch, while others are designed to target one species.[15]

All of these substances are used to kill things and they are often also toxic to humans. Surprise!

There are more than 9,700 types of pesticides in use today. Research shows that a typical boxed breakfast cereal contains residues from more than 30 of these substances. Even though each individual pesticide may be within its legal limit and deemed "safe," again, the cumulative effects and effects of these chemicals in combination with each other is unknown.[3] These compounds also have not been studied directly in people.[16]

Monsanto is one of the world's largest pesticide and herbicide producers. They also make and sell the GMO seeds that are engineered to resist the chemicals "murderous" effects. Convenient, no?

Approximately one billion pounds of Monsanto's herbicide RoundUp are used in the U.S. every year, and 56 billion pounds worldwide. RoundUp contains the controversial and toxic chemical glyphosate. Glyphosate has been registered as a pesticide since 1974.[17] It is believed most people have glyphosate in their systems due to the widespread use of RoundUp.[18]

Research shows RoundUp and other pesticides cause neurological disorders including cognitive decline, poor motor function in infants, Parkinson's, thyroid and kidney disorders, and many cancers including breast, ovarian, thyroid, prostate, and non-Hodgkin's lymphoma.[18,19] Glyphosate was recently deemed a probable carcinogen by the World Health Organization.[20]

Researchers theorize that RoundUp disrupts the normal functioning of white blood cells, causing dysfunction in the immune system and leading to illness. Data also reveals that exposure to RoundUp can potentially alter human hormones, leading to obesity, heart problems, and diabetes.[17]

A 2016 study showed glyphosate could bind to toxic metals, creating a new compound that is transported more easily in the environment and is more toxic than glyphosate itself. The behavioral effects of glyphosate were much more pronounced when it acted as this new substance.[21]

Glyphosate destroys a wide variety of pathogenic organisms and, like antibiotics, they also kill "good guys." Which makes sense, right? Researchers found that the heavy use of glyphosate has destroyed milkweed, the plant monarch butterflies need to reproduce and survive as a species, which has led to an 81 percent decrease in the monarch butterfly population.[17]

The "killer" ingredient has also recently been detected in the air and rain.[17]

When GMO technology was first introduced, chemical companies claimed it would *reduce* chemical use, but annual herbicide use has actually *increased* by over 500 million pounds. For every pound less of insecticide used, farmers actually used four pounds *more* herbicides.[17]

How well is it even working? Some plants are now becoming resistant to RoundUp, and overuse of the product has led to some nearly impossible to kill "super weeds."[17]

There is more about Monsanto in the Government chapter.

Secret Flavor Ingredients

"Secret flavor" ingredients are often referred to as "natural flavors," which is one of the most frequently used ingredients on food labels, right behind sugar and salt.[3]

These "natural flavors" are not always so "natural" however. Some of these flavor mixtures contain more than 100 substances. Examples of "secret flavor" ingredients are synthetic chemicals including the solvent propylene glycol, the preservative BHA, and products derived from genetically modified organisms.[4]

Sadly, ingredients such as these so called "natural flavors" are what have made the term "natural" in relation to food products virtually meaningless. This has added to the confusion about nutrition. Thanks, guys!

Trans Fat

Trans fat is a man-made fat created in a lab. Scientists attached hydrogen atoms to unsaturated fat, thus "saturating" it with hydrogen atoms and making it structurally similar to saturated fat.

This "test-tube" fat was meant to be a healthier alternative to, but, turned out to be even worse than saturated fat. Trans fat, also called "trans-fatty acids," both raises your LDL ("bad") cholesterol and lowers your HDL ("good") cholesterol. A diet laden with trans fat increases the risk of heart disease, the leading killer of men and women.

A form of trans fat, known as partially hydrogenated oil, is still found in a variety of processed food products.[22]

Organic Solutions

"Organic" is a term that's regulated by the USDA. Organic produce can't be treated with conventional pesticides and must be grown in nearly pesticide-free soil. For these reasons, organic fruits and vegetables have much lower pesticide residues.

To be sold as organic, livestock must meet several criteria:

- Be fed only organic, vegetarian feed
- Not be fed meat from other slaughtered animals (a common component of conventional livestock feed)
- Not be treated with any antibiotics or hormones or treated with radiation
- Living conditions allow for exercise and outdoor access

The USDA can inspect farms for compliance, and it's believed the vast majority of organic farmers follow these practices.[3]

Organic Problems

As with everything, organic foods have some drawbacks. Organic farming can be more labor intensive. Therefore, food often costs more. There are also variations in the nutrition and quality of organic foods. Although research suggests that some organic foods have more nutrients, organic practices aren't always 100 percent sustainable or "green." However, they are usually "greener" than non-organic farming.[3]

Some organic farmers also have concerns. The regulations and potential penalties involved in organic certification and the legal implications of finding *anything* out of compliance make the practice prohibitive for some farmers. Some farmers are looking at opting out of organic certification but still processing their foods as close to the organic equivalent as possible. Higher farming and production standards and consumers able to trust those who supply their food would be a dramatic improvement from where we are now.

Also, perhaps we need another word aside from "organic." "Natural" would be my preference. However, since the food industry has essentially made the term "natural" meaningless in terms of how "natural" a food is, alternate terms are needed to indicate when a food is truly "natural."

I prefer the term "unadulterated," which means "having no added substances," or "minimally processed" (since even cooking is considered "processing"). The U.S. food supply is definitely "dirty" in many ways, so the newer term "clean eating" also works.

DIY: Do It Yourself

Grow your own! Gardening is fun, inexpensive, delicious, and you know exactly what was done to the food you put into your precious body.

Buy Local

Buying from local farmers' markets ensures fresh produce. It also reduces the wasted fuel, pollution, and greenhouse gases created by long-haul shipping. Buying local also provides an opportunity to ask the farmer about the methods they used to produce the food.[3]

Conclusion

Consuming too much processed food is problematic for several reasons. These foods do not have the nutrients our bodies need *and* contain harmful substances. Our bodies will continue to break if this cycle doesn't stop. Those benefitting including the pharmaceutical, insurance, and others in the "disease management" system, and the adulterated food manufacturers, will continue to grow and profit and have an ever deepening resolve to continue and support it. We, the public, may one day literally be too sick and tired to fight back.

Humans have a history of not treading respectfully or lightly enough when it comes to our food, bodies, and planet. History continues to tell us that thoughtless actions usually come back to slap us—and our health—in the face. That is certainly true with regard to processed food. In addition, it is likely that we have only begun to see the negative effects of processed food, and that more will be discovered as time goes on.

Food should nourish, sustain, and heal us—not entertain us, cause cravings for more, make us sick, or gain excessive weight.

Manipulating or "adulterating" food for profit is unhealthy and unethical. These methods are getting more attention and push-back from consumers and the public at large, but harmful and unhealthy practices are still being widely used. There are, of course, natural alternatives to harsh and harmful farming and food production methods.

Buying, growing, and consuming whole, minimally processed, and ethically produced food will help get unwanted substances out of food and the environment by sending a clear message to the food industry that we don't support the abuse of our food, bodies, and environment.

It is theoretically possible for the industry to convert their unhealthy food production methods to healthier ones — because, ultimately, they just want our money. In other words, if we consumers persist, we can find our way back to truly "natural" foods.[20]

Chapter Eight

Research: In Defense of Nutrition

"Problems cannot be solved at the same level of awareness that created them."
– *Albert Einstein*

Changing society's philosophy about nutrition will require the availability of and reliance on quality research.

Some of the negative attitudes about nutrition are:

- "Nutrition is quackery"
- "Nutrition is unproven"
- "It's a waste of time and money"
- "You need these pills or you might die"
- "Natural remedies don't work"
- "We can't afford it"
- "This problem is not caused by diet"
- "Nutrition won't fix this"

The truth is that science often rebuts these arguments.

Nutritional solutions are not a waste of time and money, as we spend a lot of time and money now reacting to problems, mostly by way of surgery and pharmaceuticals. Many illnesses could be treated and prevented with natural remedies including nutrition education.

We don't *need* powerful man-created medications that are meant to treat symptoms and lead to other health problems. Our current path is unsustainable. So not only *can* we do it, we *must* do it.

Even though data exists proving that natural solutions work, we need more. However, who will fund it? Vegetable farmers? Unfortunately, those profiting, including the pharmaceutical, pesticide and "junk" food industries are funding most research today. As a result, there is now a disparity between research for profitable, disease-dependent solutions, and those that save lives and reduce costs.

The Scientific Method

The scientific method is a "method of procedure that has characterized natural science since the 17th century, consisting in systematic observation, measurement, and experiment, and the formulation, testing, and modification of hypotheses."[1]

The first step of the scientific method is to make an observation and ask questions about it. The next step is to formulate and propose an explanation, called a "hypothesis."

Experiments are then performed to test this hypothesis. It is critical that these experiments provide objective results that can be measured and *repeated* with the same results.

Based upon repeated and successful testing, a theory can be developed. Now, the word "theory" doesn't mean the same in scientific circles as it does in common usage. Generally, when people use the word "theory," they mean something closer to "hypothesis," an untested explanation for some observation. In science, however, a "theory" is an explanation based on a compilation of many experiments and repeated results.

If most of the results support the original hypothesis, a theory is established. A theory must be continually supported by new, sound evidence for it to remain in place as the best-known confirmation of a hypothesis.

A well-designed study is one of the main keys to success in science and to finding the true answer to a question.

There is no room for personal opinion in scientific research except to form a hypothesis and comment on conclusions, and then, only after data is collected and recorded. The data must be allowed to "speak" in an uninhibited manner.

To account for any bias on the investigators part, study results are interpreted in a peer-review system which is an evaluation of scientific, academic, or professional work by others working in the same field. In science, bias can still occur, but the system is designed to limit it as much as possible.

Caution should be exercised when a single study finds new results. Experiments must be repeated and similar results found to ensure the new results were not a fluke or based on a flawed study.

If the scientific method is adhered to, science should rarely be controversial. In short, the scientific method is a way to answer a question to the best of human ability.

Keeping Research Honest

As I said, much of today's research is being funded by financially interested parties. Data shows researchers often feel pressure to find an outcome that pleases the funder. This affects the study's results.[2,3] When there is bias or an agenda to find a certain outcome, the scientific method simply does *not* work.

In a review of 168 industry-funded studies, 156 of them—a whopping 93 percent—reported results that favored the funders' interests. The studies involved ranged from pharmaceuticals and medical devices to weight loss aids and sugary drinks.[4]

The Blame Game

Quality research for balanced solutions is often lacking, and what does exist is often controversial. Many scientists and their research results are being questioned, sadly, often because their findings contradict the goals of the profiteers.

Dietitians are sometimes blamed for being a part of our public nutrition problems. Some think we obediently recommend a diet based on what is dictated to us, by the USDA via their Food Guide for example.

Let me add some clarity to this myth. A dietitian is someone who completed nutrition training in a qualifying didactic program which was either a four-year or an advanced degree program. Dietitians are highly trained to find, decipher, understand, and scrutinize data using the scientific method.

At U.C. Davis, one of the most well-regarded didactic programs in the world, students, including me, evaluated piles of research from reliable, well-designed, well-conducted studies done on large populations by trained scientists who were looking for *answers*. My classmates and I learned how to formulate healthy diet plans based on best practices from around the globe.

Dietitians are highly educated and qualified scientists trained to disseminate accurate and current nutrition information based on *facts*. Blaming scientists, the research they do, or others working for solutions such as teachers, which will be covered later, misses the real problem.

After all, who has more to gain from inaccurate information: scientists, dietitians, and teachers, or big money makers like the pharmaceutical, pesticide, and "junk" food industries?

To find a trusted source, consider whether the main motivation is to provide information and keep public trust or to maximize financial gain.

The healing, preventative, and cost-effective abilities of natural solutions, including nutritional ones, have been proven. Interestingly much of this research is done in other countries, where finding profitable pharmacologic solutions is less of a priority than it is in the U.S.

However, plenty of data does exist. Here is some of that research.

Research Samples

Allergies and Asthma

- Research suggests links between folate and allergies and asthma. In a study funded by the National Institutes of Health, researchers reviewed medical data from 8,083 patients from a 2005-2006 study where serum folate levels and the levels of antibodies present in allergic reactions were measured. Higher levels of folate were linked to lower antibody levels, fewer reports of allergies, less wheezing, and a lower likelihood of developing asthma. Lower levels of folate were related to a 40 percent increase in the likelihood of an attack. The researchers concluded that additional research was needed to confirm these early findings and to understand the mechanisms involved.[5]
- Study results showed a reduced risk of asthma by 50 percent in children who increased their intake of whole grains and fish.[6]

Attention Deficit Disorder (ADD)

- Study results have shown that artificial food coloring and benzoate preservatives have a negative effect on the behavior of children.[7]
- Fifty-nine of 78 children with hyperactive behavior placed on an elimination diet had improved behavior.[8]
- Study results have shown three percent of gifted children had borderline hypoglycemic conditions and allergies. When combined with sensitivity and intensity, this leads to behavior that mimics ADD symptoms.[9]
- Certain foods and food additives are common causes of ADD in children. In one study, almost 75 percent of study subjects had an adverse reaction when exposed to these triggers. The children reacted to many foods, dyes, and preservatives. Results demonstrated a beneficial effect of eliminating reactive foods and artificial colors in children with ADD. The researchers concluded that dietary factors may play a significant role in the

etiology of the majority of children with ADD.[10]

- Scientists conducted a randomized six-week, double-blind, placebo-controlled trial of 44 outpatient children who had been diagnosed with ADD. The study was conducted in order to see if using the mineral zinc in addition to methylphenidate or Ritalin could alleviate the symptoms of ADD more than drugs alone. There have been other studies that have found zinc alone helps reduce ADD symptoms. Zinc plays a role in regulating the brain chemicals melatonin and dopamine. Melatonin affects sleep patterns. Dopamine affects many things including attention. The results of this study showed a reduction in ADD symptoms in both groups of children. At six weeks, the improvement in the group supplemented with zinc was greater than that of the placebo group. The improvement seen in the behavior of both groups was similar, but significant improvement was seen and reported on the Teacher Parent Rating Scale in the group supplemented with zinc. This study substantiates the hypothesis that there is a relationship between zinc and the treatment of ADD symptoms.[11]

- A clinical trial was performed on children between ages 8 and 10 who were found to be iron deficient. Iron deposits are found in areas of the brain where dopamine is regulated. Dopamine levels affect concentration and attention. It was hypothesized that iron deficiencies might lead to imbalances of dopamine which, in turn, would lead to attention deficits. The results of the study showed a significant improvement in the test scores of iron-deficient children after iron supplementation, showing a strong correlation between attention and iron deficiency.[12]

Bipolar Disorder

- Supplements of omega-3 fatty acids can have a positive effect on bipolar disorder. In one such study, omega-3 helped stabilize the condition of patients with this disorder. A different dose lowered patients' aggression.[13]

- See also, *"Mental Illness"*

Blood Pressure

- There may be a link between vitamin C and blood pressure. In one study, researchers concluded that those with the highest levels of vitamin C had the lowest blood pressure.[14]
- Study results have shown that green and brown algae have strong anticoagulant or blood-thinning activity, suggesting the potential for the treatment of blood clots.[15]
- Scientific evidence has shown that many nutrients and plants including omega-3 fatty acids, hibiscus, stevia, calcium, and Coenzyme Q10 are beneficial in treating high blood pressure.[16]

Bone Density

- Researchers discovered that genistein, a nutrient found in soybeans and peanuts, may help increase bone health by reducing bone loss in women with low bone density. One such study concluded that genistein has positive effects on bone mineral density.[17]
- Other nutritional therapies with notable preliminary evidence in the treatment of low bone density include calcium, vitamin D, black tea, boron, copper, creatine, dehydroepiandrosterone (DHEA), gamma linolenic acid, horsetail, red clover, soy, tamarind, and vitamin K.[17]

Cancer

- Data shows fruit and vegetable consumption can prevent cancer. The following image is from one of my UC-Davis clinical nutrition courses taken in 2006. This table shows a correlation between consuming fruits and vegetables and a lower risk of all types of cancer. For example, in lung cancer, 24 out of 25 studies show a relationship between consumption of fruits and vegetables and a reduced risk of lung cancer.

Epidemiologic Studies of Fruit and Vegetable Intake and Cancer Risk

Cancer Site	Number of Studies (Protective)	Inverse Association
		(P<0.05)
All Sites, except prostate	156	128
Stomach	19	17
Colorectal	27	20
Bladder	5	3
Cervix	8	7
Ovary	4	3
Breast	14	8
Prostate	14	4
Lung	25	24
Larynx	4	4
Oral Cavity, Pharynx	9	9
Esophagus	16	15
Pancreas	11	9

- A similar graph in that same UC-Davis course showed that increased meat consumption correlated to *higher* rates of cancer.[18]
- Study results have shown that citrus components tangeretin and nobiletin can stop cancerous cell growth and significantly suppress cancer cell proliferation. Based on these results, it has been determined that citrus can be an effective anti-cancer agent.[19]
- Mushrooms have been shown to have cancer-fighting abilities, including anti-tumor effects.[20,21]
- A long-term study was done on 48 men age 60 and up who underwent treatment for prostate cancer. All of the men had rising prostate specific antigen (PSA) levels after treatment. Increased PSA levels are associated with prostate cancer. During the six-year follow-up, men who drank pomegranate juice had lower PSA levels than those who had stopped drinking the juice.[22]
- Study results have shown that the consumption of polyphenon E, an ingredient in green tea, led to cancer regression and tumor reduction in significant numbers of patients — over 50 percent of participants in one study.[23]

- Curcumin, derived from the roots of *Curcuma longa*, a member of the ginger family and a major component of the spice turmeric, is one of the hottest plant polyphenol extracts being researched today. In the past 10 years alone, there have been more than 4,600 scientific papers published on curcumin. Many of these studies suggest that this compound could be useful in the prevention and treatment of a wide spectrum of medical conditions and physiologic processes, including cancer, inflammatory diseases, cystic fibrosis, and Alzheimer's disease.[24,25]

Cognition and Memory

- Low blood levels of vitamin D may be associated with increased odds of cognitive impairment.[26]
- Study results have shown that a vitamin C deficiency in the first weeks of life results in impaired neuronal development and a decrease in memory in guinea pigs.[27]

Depression

- Study results have shown that tyrosine, phenylalanine, and tryptophan can alleviate depression.[28]
- Consistent epidemiological evidence, particularly for depression, suggests an association between measures of diet quality and mental health across multiple populations and age groups that do not appear to be explained by other demographic or lifestyle factors.[29]

Eating Disorders

- In a study published in the *Archives of General Psychiatry*, patients with a history of bulimia nervosa who were given an amino acid supplement without tryptophan experienced a relapse more often than those who were given a balanced amino acid supplement.[30]

Health Education

- Experts reviewed the literature to assess empirical research about health literacy, health behavior, and health status outcomes. They found most programs were focused only on health literacy.

The researchers found a lack of evidence supporting the effectiveness of focusing on health literacy alone and found comprehensive health education that included a focus on behavior changes and skill development led to more positive health outcomes.

The researchers concluded, "We recommend that comprehensive school health education serve as the standard for advancing personal health and health outcomes. We recommend that elementary, secondary, and higher education institutions be charged with the objective to provide comprehensive school health education intervention to advance personal health, community health, and concomitantly moderate national healthcare expenditures."[31]

Healthcare Cost Savings

- According to a report by the National Academy of Sciences Institute of Medicine (IOM), receiving nutritional therapy is cost effective. Dietitians can help people manage conditions such as high blood pressure, high cholesterol, diabetes, and kidney and heart problems.
- In a study done by the Department of Veterans Affairs, more than half of the people who received nutrition counseling from a dietitian lowered their cholesterol and no longer needed cholesterol medication. Nutrition therapy ended up saving the healthcare system $60,000 per year in prescription drug costs.

On a national level, according to the IOM report, such savings can translate into millions. If Medicare beneficiaries with high blood pressure received nutrition therapy, healthcare costs over a five-year period could be cut by an estimated $52 million to $167 million for hypertension alone. Findings such as this led the IOM report's authors to conclude that Medicare should cover physician-ordered nutrition counseling.[32]

Learning, Behavior, Grades and Attendance

- Children who participated in the Universal School Breakfast Program performed better in school. Children at nutritional risk who received breakfast at school had an increase in grades and decrease in problems related to attendance and behavior. Participation in a school breakfast program enhanced daily nutrient intake, which was associated with significant improvement in math grades and behavior.[33]
- Skipping breakfast was associated with decreased cognitive performance (e.g., alertness, attention, memory, processing of complex visual display, problem solving) among students.
- Lack of adequate consumption of specific foods, such as fruits and vegetables, was associated with lower grades among students.
- Deficits of specific nutrients (i.e., vitamins A, B6, B12, C, folate, iron, zinc, and calcium) were associated with lower grades and higher rates of absenteeism and tardiness among students.
- Hunger due to insufficient food intake was associated with lower grades, higher rates of absenteeism, repeating a grade, and an inability to focus among students.[34]

Medical School Nutrition Education

- Ninety-nine of 106 accredited U.S. medical schools surveyed required some form of nutrition education. However, only 32 schools required a separate nutrition course. On average, medical school students received only 24 hours of nutrition instruction.
- Only 40 medical schools required the minimum number of instructional hours recommended by the National Academy of Sciences, which is 25.
- Approximately 90 percent of instructors expressed the need for additional nutrition instruction.[35]

Mental Illness

- The treatments for mental illness, including depression, anxiety, and bipolar disorder, are primarily pharmacotherapy and psychotherapy. However, these treatments fail to address the entirety of the disease burden. This suggests that additional strategies are needed to prevent and treat mental disorders. Consistent data suggests the use of dietary and nutraceutical interventions in mental disorders are effective. Nutraceuticals, including n-3 fatty acids, folate, S-adenosylmethionine, N-acetyl cysteine, and probiotics, among others, are a promising avenue for future research.

A recently published intervention trial provides preliminary clinical evidence that dietary interventions in clinically diagnosed populations are feasible and can provide significant benefit.[29]

Nutrition Education

- A study done by the United States Department of Agriculture found that 69 percent of participants in a nutrition education program had an increase in nutrition knowledge, and 61 percent had an increased ability to select low-cost, nutritious foods. The entire group showed an overall improvement in their consumption of fruits and vegetables. Adults in the program showed a 91 percent improvement in consumption of nutritious foods, and 88 percent improved their nutrition practices. At the start of the program, only 20 percent of the adult participants reported consuming at least half of the daily recommended amount of fruits and vegetables. At the end of the program, this increased to 41 percent. The researchers concluded that educational opportunities and resources for nutrition education need to be increased.[36]
- School garden program participants increased their consumption of fruits and vegetables. Students who participated in a Berkeley, CA, school garden program ate 1.5 more fruit and vegetable servings a day than those who did not participate in the program.[37]
- Research shows that between 40 and 50 hours of nutrition education may be necessary to be effective.

A massive study was done of more than 1,000 classrooms in which four model curricula were tested on 30,000 students in grades four through seven. Program-specific knowledge increased substantially during the first 15 hours of classroom instruction, but general knowledge, practices, and attitudes did not increase to their maximal levels until after 40 to 50 hours of classroom instruction. The study focused on one year of instruction. There were even better results when the information was built on in following years.

However, the researchers found that nutrition and dietary behavior topics only consume a median of 3.4 hours in elementary schools, 4.2 hours in middle schools, and 5.9 hours in high schools.

A typical school year includes about 1,000 hours of instruction. Since Health Education topics may need 40 to 50 hours of time to have optimal effects, teachers may be hard pressed to include everything they are required to instruct if other subjects outside of the standard curriculum require comparable amounts of time. Thus, some of the hours may need to come from other school venues.[38] Suggestions for how to do this are discussed in the Education chapter.

Research Conflict of Interest

- The *American Journal of Psychiatry* took an in-depth look at the financial conflict of interest in clinical trials; research that it is believed had never been done before, and found a greater likelihood that the results were favorable to the source of the funding. The researchers examined the funding source and author financial conflict of interest in all clinical trials published in psychiatry journals between 2001 and 2003. They found that, of 397 clinical trials studied, 239 (60 percent) reported receiving funding from a pharmaceutical company or other interested party. 187 studies (50 percent) included at least one author with a reported financial conflict of interest. Among the 162 of 187 studies that were examined, it was found that those that reported conflict of interest were about five times more likely to report positive results among the pharmaceutical industry-funded studies.

The researchers concluded that author conflict of interest was prevalent in psychiatric clinical trials and led to "a greater likelihood of reporting a drug to be superior to placebo."[3]

Rheumatoid Arthritis

- Accumulating research evidence suggests that individual dietary factors and patterns might be implicated in the risk of development of rheumatoid arthritis (RA). Overall, a Western-type diet high in energy intake (calories), total and saturated fat, refined carbohydrates and sugar, an unbalanced ratio of n-3 to n-6 fatty acids, and low in fiber and antioxidants, might increase the risk of RA both directly through increasing inflammation and indirectly through increasing insulin resistance and obesity.

  On the other hand consumption of long-chain omega-3 polyunsaturated fatty acids derived from fish and fish oil, is associated with a reduced risk of RA, probably due to the anti-inflammatory properties of omega-3s. The Mediterranean Diet, which is rich in plant-based foods such as whole grains, legumes, fruit, vegetables, and extra-virgin olive oil, and limits red meat consumption, might have the potential to reduce the risk of RA.

  Further research on RA susceptibility will allow for more specific dietary recommendations.[39]

Schizophrenia

- A Danish study showed that better prognoses for schizophrenic patients strongly correlate with living in a country where there is a high consumption of omega-3 fatty acids. The omegas have been shown to help depressive patients and can also be used to treat schizophrenia. Furthermore, omega supplements taken on a daily basis help both healthy individuals and schizophrenic patients maintain a balanced mood and improved blood circulation.

- Consumption of refined sugar resulted in a decline in the state of mind for schizophrenic patients.
- Diet may be able to predict schizophrenia and depression.
- Schizophrenic patients have been found to have an impaired ability to make serotonin which can come from amino acids. High doses of glycine have been shown to reduce some symptoms of schizophrenia such as social withdrawal, emotional flatness, and apathy, that don't respond to today's medications. A 1996 clinical trial revealed that glycine could be given to schizophrenic patients without producing adverse side effects.[40]

Weight Loss

- African mango supplementation resulted in one study's participants losing an average of 28 pounds each. The participants also had lowered cholesterol and blood sugar. Participants who did not take the supplement had no notable weight loss. Earlier studies also found the same result.[41]

Conclusion

Research clearly shows that natural and preventative measures work, yet they are largely being disregarded. Let's choose a new path, one that relies on the scientific method to solve problems as it was designed to do.

More research can be found on Pubmed.gov. A summary of the study, including the results, can be found in the free "Abstract" section. PubMed has also begun listing potential conflicts of interest on some studies. This is progress!

Let the good data flow and it will overpower the noise.

Chapter Nine

The Brain: It's All Related

"It's bizarre that the produce manager is more important to my children's health than the pediatrician."
– Meryl Streep

Nutrition affects our bodies and *our brains*. Mental disorders account for four out of 10 leading causes of disability in developed countries, including the U.S. There has been an increase in the number of mental health disorders in developed countries due to the deterioration of the Western diet.[1]

Many patients who have mental disorders are found to have nutrient deficiencies. However, very few mentally ill patients are treated naturally. Instead, they're given powerful medications that often cause side effects including a dulled personality, reduced emotions, memory loss, and tremors.[1,2]

Nutrition has been proven to play a role in mental disorders including addiction, anxiety, attention deficit disorder (ADD), autism, bipolar disease, dementia, depression, eating disorders, obsessive-compulsive disorder, and schizophrenia.[1,3]

Diet intervention can be used to treat and sometimes even *cure* mental disorders. However, as researchers have reported, nutritional therapies are a "long-forgotten method of treatment" in mental disorders because the drug companies have no interest in pursuing something they cannot patent or own.[1]

Many nutritional studies conducted in the 1970s and 1980s looked at how nutrition may play a role in disorders of the brain, but much of the research was dropped due to underfunding.[1]

Attention Disorders

Attention Deficit Disorder (ADD), now often referred to as Attention Deficit Hyperactivity Disorder (ADHD), is a subject close to my heart, as the many children suffering from these disorders inspired me to go back to college and study nutrition. I felt strongly then and now that diet is involved in these disorders, and the data continues to confirm this. Children do not suffer from a Ritalin deficiency after all.

The symptoms of Attention Deficit Disorder include difficulty concentrating, inability to sit still, irritability, hyperactivity, impulsiveness, and mood swings. There is no known cause, although emerging evidence suggests it relates to chemical imbalances in the brain.

The original name ADD was expanded to include hyperactivity, hence the "H" in ADHD. Now, potential diagnoses have expanded to include ADHD with residuals, meaning bipolar symptoms. The name keeps getting longer and more complex as more is discovered. Basically, the medical community does not truly understand these disorders but simply give them names and expanding acronyms. For simplicity, I will continue to refer to this "disorder" as ADD.

ADD is the most commonly diagnosed mental disorder in children. According to the Centers for Disease Control and Prevention (CDC), 10 percent of children have been diagnosed with this disorder.[4,5]

It is likely not a coincidence that kids today are eating more "junk" food, more poor-quality food, and more food on-the-go than any other generation in this country's history.

Many symptoms of ADD are identical to symptoms caused by poor nutrition. For example, studies have implicated food sensitivities, food allergies, fatty acids, and an excess of food additives and refined sugars in ADD.[6]

In fact, data has shown diet interventions have a better than 70 percent success rate in treating ADD,[7] but very few patients ever receive nutritional treatment. Instead, millions of children are being prescribed powerful stimulants, which aim to stimulate inactive areas in the brain and other medications.[8]

Their educations suffer too as children cannot focus, pay attention, or learn because their bodies are chemically out of balance. It is heart-wrenching to consider what diet-induced imbalances are doing to children's small, growing bodies.

The "Attention Deficit" drug market is valued at $4 billion annually and is one of the most rapidly growing drug markets in the U.S.[9,10]

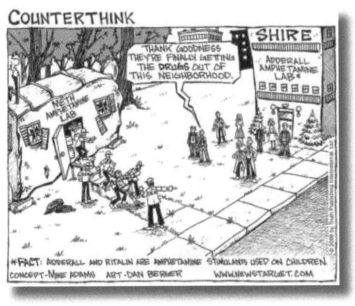

Amphetamines are most often prescribed for ADD. These drugs have a similar chemical structure to and the same addictive qualities of cocaine.[11] Despite being among the most prescribed medications, however, these drugs are not particularly effective. Of those treated with stimulant medication, 42 percent do not respond as intended, and some even show increased behavior problems.[12]

Some of the side effects of amphetamine medications include insomnia, decreased appetite, stomachache, headache, dizziness, sadness, crying, picking at the skin, irritability, nightmares, tics, weight loss, reduced growth, agitation, anxiousness, psychosis, Tourette's syndrome, cognitive impairment, hypertension, hyperthyroidism, cardiovascular problems, glaucoma, and fatal liver damage.[12]

Antidepressants, also commonly prescribed for ADD, cause side effects such as constipation, drowsiness, increased blood pressure, blurred vision, dry mouth, hyperactivity, nausea, facial rash, feeling "spaced out," cardiac toxicity, and sudden death.[12]

Anti-hypertensives used to treat ADD cause side effects such as sedation, irritability, headaches, stomachaches, cardiac changes, and drops in blood pressure and heart rate.[12]

There is ample data proving the effectiveness of nutritional remedies in treating mental disorders and illnesses such as ADD. Nutritional treatments are milder, cheaper, often more effective, and have fewer detrimental "side effects" than drugs.

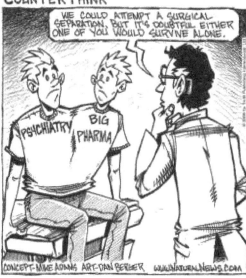

Dangerous medications should be used as a *last*, not a *first* resort.

In addition, prescribing medications for a disorder we do not understand sends the wrong message to our children; that drugs are the answer.

Chapter Ten

Education: A Primary Solution

"Knowledge is power."
– Sir Francis Bacon

There is no doubt we have a health crisis in the U.S. More than 70 percent of Americans over the age of 20 and roughly 20 percent of children are overweight or obese.[1] One in four school-age children now has diabetes or prediabetes.[2] There are ever-increasing occurrences of lifestyle diseases, including rheumatoid arthritis, cancer, and heart disease. Many of these and other health epidemics can be attributed to poor diet due to a lack of proper nutrition education.[3,4,5]

Enter public education. The not-for-profit public school system is an ideal venue to deliver desperately needed accurate nutrition information, the antidote to help heal and prevent many of our nation's plagues. Currently, this opportunity is being passed over as we continue to put education, including nutrition education, "on the back burner."

There *is* a plethora of for-profit, biased information available for what ails us including the marketing of medications, and plenty of diet books that claim to have discovered the latest miracle cure. We *don't have* sufficient public information networks to provide honest, comprehensive information about nutrition. Sadly, most people cannot tell the difference between for-profit information (usually biased) and not-for-profit (less biased).

Diagnosing the Problems

The current educational system is struggling and often failing to meet many of its academic requirements, so simply adding more content will not work.[6] In order to fix any problem we must look at it comprehensively.

There is no shortage of people who have ideas about how to "fix" public education; but these are often *inexperienced* people on the outside looking in who do not truly understand what is really going on.

Because the U.S. public school funding model is based on local property taxes, more funding is funneled to schools with students from higher income levels, and less to those with students from lower income levels. This translates into lower test scores in low-income areas.

Teachers are often blamed for the problems in education. They are continually asked to try this or that "new and improved" method, take on more duties, and "teach to the test."

"Teaching used to be a creative and fun way to make a living," said a 35-year elementary school teacher and former colleague, "but now, there is so much pressure on and demonization of teachers, that the joy of learning has been lost in the pursuit of test scores."

On top of that, many students, teachers, and staff members are dealing with excessive stress, anxiety, and exhaustion.

Most teachers I know feel there are inadequate resources available to meet the needs of all of their students, especially in at-risk areas where students need more resources and attention. Most of us try anyway, often at the expense of our own pocketbooks, private lives, and health.

There are more than 15,000 school districts in the U.S., and the many layers of state and federal departments that regulate them add to an already bureaucratic-heavy system. Teachers and students are doing more than ever. Class sizes are larger than most people think is appropriate. Not surprisingly, the teaching profession lacks new candidates, as many do not want the relatively low pay for the heavy burden that now comes with being a public school teacher.[7]

Many children today either aren't learning effectively or drop out of school altogether. This leads to lower education levels and limited job opportunities. Many children without an education end up incarcerated. In fact, one out of every 31 people in the U.S. is now in the U.S. correctional system. The U.S. has five percent of the world's population but houses 25 percent of its inmates.[8] An individual without a proper education is more likely to end up in jail or on welfare.

We *have* to adjust our priorities.

Those without an adequate education generally also lack access to health resources including healthy food and healthcare, adequate coping mechanisms, and basic life skills. This leads to an increased risk of depression; stress; unhealthy relationships; physical, verbal, and emotional abuse; drug abuse; perpetrating or experiencing crime and violence; incarceration; poverty; homelessness; illness; and premature death. This is unacceptable, inhumane, expensive, and *is solvable*.

Education is not a luxury. It is a necessity. If we remain on our current path, more members of our society will become sick, less educated, and productive. The result will be spending more resources (which cost money) to solve problems that could have been prevented through education.

Preventative measures such as education can help reverse cycles of failure. However, a change in *philosophy* is required. Immeasurable costs including financial, emotional and security related ones, would be saved through adequate implementation of preventative programs such as health and nutrition education. First, we must collectively decide that failure is no longer an option.

Nutrition Education

I hear people say, "Everyone knows how to eat healthy, they just don't want to." Unfortunately, they don't. Since most people don't even receive a *basic* nutrition education, not everyone "knows how to eat healthy." This is abundantly clear when you look at the health of our society.

Food is the base of our body chemistry and determines our body and brain function. Sadly, most people are untrained "chemists" performing important experiments on their own bodies.

Research consistently shows that schools with a coordinated nutrition program provide a more focused message about the importance of nutrition and have better results. Even though these comprehensive nutritional programs lead to improved health, learning, and educational outcomes, very few of these programs exist in the U.S.[9,10]

The majority of public school nutrition education focuses on the USDA Food Guide. Less than half of schools providing nutrition education thoroughly cover topics such as the relationship between diet and health which is what research shows really works.[10] Even though the USDA Food Guide is predominantly covered in classrooms that offer nutrition education, only two percent of U.S. children ages 2 to 19 eats a diet consistent with it.[11]

Research reveals that many of the instructional materials and techniques used to teach nutrition are ineffective. Studies also show the amount of time devoted to the topic is not sufficient to create dietary changes.[12]

Research also shows that for healthy behavioral changes including shopping, buying, preparing, and eating healthy food, a minimum of 40 to 50 hours of instruction are needed.[9,12]

Obviously, finding 40 to 50 hours in a school curriculum to cover nutrition could be challenging, but there are *ways* to do it if the *will* to do it exists. For instance, nutrition could be embedded into other curriculum areas such as science, math, and English, and in school garden programs and comprehensive Health Classes.

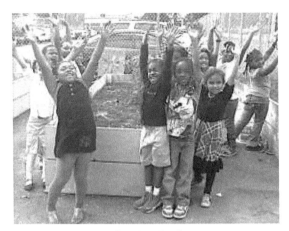

Planting Seeds

Outdoor Education Programs: A.K.A. "Garden Class"

One approach to providing comprehensive nutrition education is via the implementation of school gardens, also known as "outdoor classrooms." I have personally managed and taught in school gardens in grades pre-kindergarten through 12th.

Outdoor classrooms provide real-world, hands-on opportunities to teach multiple subjects including history, math, science, health, and nutrition.

Many U.S. public elementary schools have school gardens, but integrating them into the core curriculum can be a challenge. These outdoor educational programs are highly successful *if* they have an individual or group dedicated to facilitating them. I was one of those people, and it worked!

Life Lab, The Center for Ecoliteracy, and The Edible Schoolyard are among the numerous educational organizations that utilize school gardens as functioning classrooms and see them as a place where science, nature, and nutrition can be taught with the right program focus and intention.

Life Lab promotes experiential learning for people of all ages through field trips, children's camps, and teacher workshops in Santa Cruz and Watsonville, CA.[13]

The Center for Ecoliteracy provides resources and support to school garden programs "at multiple levels of scale, with local, regional, state, and national programs."[14]

The Edible Schoolyard in Berkeley, CA, incorporates classroom instruction, gardening, and cooking into the studies of math, science, history, and reading, and the data shows it works.[15]

Outdoor education programs are not only effective but are also *cost effective*. Garden supplies are inexpensive and often donated by a supportive community. The produce grown by the students can be used in the cafeteria and for classroom tastings as is done in successful programs such as The Edible Schoolyard in Berkeley.[16]

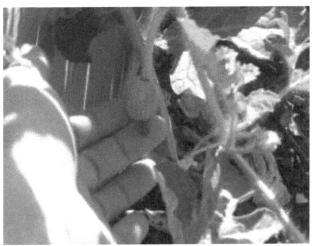

Baby Watermelon

The data is in. Outdoor nutrition educational programs work! Research results consistently prove the effectiveness of outdoor education programs on nutrition and learning. In one survey, Life Lab surveyed 452 Watsonville, CA, students who participated in garden-based nutrition lessons and food tastings. The survey found that half of them were trying healthy foods such as beets, carrots, chard, kale, and tangerines for the first time. The results showed that most—more than two-thirds—of the students liked *or loved* the food they had grown and tasted.[2]

School gardening increases the willingness of children to eat a wider range of fruits and vegetables. Students who participate in garden nutritional programs eat three times more fruits and vegetables than those who do not. When children grow it, they want to eat it.[17,18]

School gardens can also have a positive effect on a child's mental health. Researchers found that just five minutes each day of an activity such as gardening can boost mood and self-esteem. School gardens can also positively impact a child's development, teach life skills, and elevate mood.[19]

"When kids get to be hands-on with food, see it growing, harvest it, that creates a connection that makes them want to try it and [they are] more likely to enjoy it. And [that] leads to lifelong changes," says Don Burgett, Executive Director of Life Lab.[2]

I have witnessed this transformation thousands of times in my own outdoor education programs.

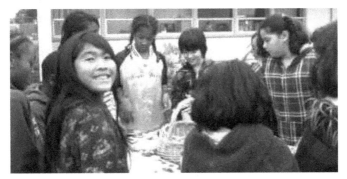

Making Salsa in the Outdoor Classroom

Nutrition Education in Health Class
Nutrition education would fit well as a part of Health Class and does

exactly that in the yearlong High School Health Class that I teach in Salinas, CA. Unfortunately, this extremely rare and very effective program is, like many other health education programs, always at risk of being cut.

Research proves that healthy students fare better on all levels of academic achievement including academic performance, education, behavior, cognitive skills, and attitudes. Healthy, successful students help build strong communities. Furthermore, all children deserve the opportunity to be healthy and successful.[20]

Most adults in the United States are not proficient in matters affecting their health. There are 75 million people in this country who have basic or below basic health literacy, which is the degree to which an individual has the capacity to process, obtain, and understand basic health information and services needed to make appropriate decisions regarding their health. It is estimated that $70 billion of our healthcare costs can be attributed to a low level of health literacy.[5]

However, focusing on health literacy alone is often not enough. For behavior changes that lead to better health outcomes, research shows that a program must include skills development as opposed to simply delivering information. A skills-based curriculum is effective as it involves students *participating* in their learning and allows opportunities for students to contextualize the information and practice the necessary skills.[21]

A quality comprehensive Health Education program teaches students to make healthy food choices, read food labels, plan meals, analyze influences on why they make specific decisions regarding nutrition (e.g., advertisements and family behaviors), and critique one's own diet. This comprehensive approach is more effective than being lectured to, just reading about, or memorizing nutrients.

There are caveats. Health Class sounds like a perfect solution to begin to tackle the ginormous problem of lack of nutrition education in this country, right? Not so fast. Yes, High School Health Class is a great place to begin to provide public nutrition education. However, Health Class, like others often considered expendable such as art and music, is regularly "on the chopping block" when it comes to school funding. In context with all of the health and other problems our society is facing, this makes zero sense, right?

Many school districts have either condensed the Health Class curriculum or eliminated Health Class altogether, and many credentialing programs no longer offer a Health Sciences Teaching Credential. This is exactly the opposite of where we should be going.

In many schools, the task of teaching Health lands on the Physical Education or Biology teachers. While they may try to do their best, they are not always qualified to delve into the nuances of nutrients or other health-related topics.

It is not uncommon for educators to be approached by guest speakers from various for-profit corporations (e.g., Frito Lay, the Dairy Council, and others) with offers to provide materials and presentations to the students. Some educators are strapped for time and resources, especially in condensed programs, and may be tempted to use this biased information.

In fact, many school districts are currently *not* meeting the requirements of the California Education Code for teaching Health.

It is the decision of the school district to determine if Health Class should be a graduation requirement. My district is one of a handful in California that has a required yearlong Health Class for graduation, and it is always at risk of being cut. Of the small number of remaining public school Health Classes in the U.S., most are only a semester long or shorter, if they exist at all.

My Health Class
My yearlong Health Class encompasses mental, emotional, social, and

physical health. Topics include healthy relationships, sexual and reproductive health, mental disorders, dealing with emotions, exercise, sleep, and, of course, nutrition. There is a course outline in Appendix B.

Our district's comprehensive Health Class regularly produces students who fondly and readily remember many activities they participated in. Memorable class activities include role plays, group projects, peer teaching, skill building activities such as refusing jelly bean "pills" at a "party," planting seeds, healthy food tastings, experimenting with "drunk goggles," sleep and food diaries, and a multitude of guest speakers, vetted by the District Health Steering Committee and the highly qualified Health Teachers who had the time and resources to do it. Some of the students' favorite speakers include those from Planned Parenthood, former addicts, and suicide counselors.

These various activities in conjunction with the relationship building that happens over the course of a year in this "Health Class family" would simply not be possible in a shortened class.

I spend approximately 180 days with the same students, teaching them healthy life skills that, frankly, most people do not have or spend a lifetime acquiring. A colleague refers to what we do as "re-parenting," which many of our students as well as members of our society need.

During the final edits of this book, our school board was tasked with voting on whether or not to cut our comprehensive Health Program in half. The public was allowed to appeal to the board by attending and speaking at the meeting or in writing. I thought about what I could say about the value of the program in under three minutes during the 20-minute public comment section at the monthly school board meeting. It would be impossible to explain in three minutes what we do in 180+ days in the Health classroom. In fact, unless one experiences it, it is impossible to comprehend all that happens in those healthy spaces throughout the year.

For several reasons, some personal ones, I chose to write to the board. I explained that we are saving and improving lives and breaking cycles. I also attached a copy of this book. I let them know it would be sad if this program was cut, and it would be especially sad to have to update this book to say this rare and stellar program was, like so many others, cut.

In addition to the other topics covered, students experience two weeks of nutrition content which is more than what most Americans get and *way better* than nothing. Also, throughout the year, I can continually build on what we covered. For instance, if I see them eating "junk" food, we have another chat about healthy eating.

Health Class is a "life class," and 10 months of life happens over the course of the school year. Throughout the year, we get to know and respect each other and discuss life events as they happen; using real-world opportunities to practice the healthy coping skills they learned about in Health Class.

Wouldn't you have liked to have that class when you were a teenager? Odds are you didn't. Neither did I. Many people, including myself, want that to change. And why not? Money? A more important class? Bologna! Think of the problems that could be solved, lives that could be bettered, and the cost to society that could be saved with more preventative programs like a yearlong Health Class. As they say, "Without our health we have nothing." Health is one of the most important classes one can take.

We will see what happens and whether or not my district holds strong and continues to support prevention and healing.

In February 2019, I went before the district school board and spoke about the value of our yearlong Health program; I even read excerpts from this book. However, despite pleas from me, students, community members, and my fellow Health teachers, the Salinas Union High School District voted to cut the yearlong Health program in half. Several board members complained about the process and lack of transparency, but it passed anyway and by only one vote. The cut was proposed as the only way to add Ethnic Studies, which was previously an elective or optional course, as a graduation requirement. The majority of families, teachers, staff and, most importantly, Health Class students adamantly disagree with the decision. The students are protesting and have even created a website, a petition, and held a small demonstration. See Appendix C for more information.

We were told by a veteran teacher and union representative that it would take families (e.g., voters) to protest strongly enough to persuade the district to look into alternatives. To which the students replied, "Why, don't our voices matter?" The problem in Salinas, and other areas, is parental involvement is minimal, so this is unlikely to happen. It is not that they don't care, as the parents and guardians I speak to are overwhelmingly in support of the yearlong Health Class. Sadly, many don't get involved mainly for cultural and economic reasons, including language barriers.

This is no doubt a devastating blow to the fight for preventative health, as this program was extremely effective and Salinas was being used as a model for wider implementation of yearlong Health Class across the state. However, I am hopeful that we will win the larger war and, via legislation or some other means, we will implement comprehensive Health education across the U.S., including Salinas. Because our society so desperately needs it, and because health education works!

Others See Value of Health Class

The Society of Health and Physical Educators, "SHAPE America," states, "Health education is a subject that is equally important—arguably, more important—than other core subjects. It is a subject that belongs in schools and that should be recognized as critical to students' education and development."[21]

The World Health Organization (WHO) stated, "An effective school health program can be one of the most cost effective investments a nation can make to simultaneously improve education and health."[22]
Students agree!

The majority of the Health students I have talked to find their yearlong Health Class interesting and helpful. My former students often tell me how much they miss Health Class, that it was their favorite class, how much they learned, how much it helped them and those around them, and some have even suggested that Health be required during every year of high school. On the other hand, former students of condensed programs (e.g., one semester or combined with other classes) usually do not have any notable memories or knowledge they can quickly access.

Several of my students have written letters of support for their yearlong Health program. Examples of these testimonials can be found in Appendix C. Student and family voices can be powerful when advocating for these vulnerable programs.

Other Frameworks for Nutrition Education

One route to comprehensive Health Education is to include it as a college entrance requirement or an "A-G" course (we health advocates refer to this as an "A through H" requirement, as H for Health – get it?). The A-G College Entrance Requirements are a sequence of high school courses that students must complete with a grade of C or better in order to be minimally eligible for admission to the University of California (UC) and California State University (CSU) systems. This would prioritize Health Class and make it much less likely to be eliminated.

There are other pathways to ensuring that comprehensive health education is provided, including through legislation, enforcement of the California Education Code, and district Wellness Policies.

School Wellness Policies

School Wellness Policies are another way to help bring nutrition and health education to schools. Districts that participate in the National School Lunch or School Breakfast Program, or any other federal Child Nutrition programs, are required by federal law to establish a Wellness Policy (WP) for all schools under its jurisdiction.

Wellness is defined as, "A healthy state of balance among multiple dimensions of wellness, including the physical, social, emotional/mental, intellectual, spiritual, environmental, and occupational."[21]

A Wellness Policy is a written document of official policies that guide a school district's efforts to establish a school environment that promotes students' health, well-being, and ability to learn by supporting healthy eating and physical activity.

A comprehensive Wellness Policy can be an important tool for parents and school districts in promoting student wellness, preventing and reducing childhood obesity, and providing assurance that school meal nutrition guidelines meet the minimum federal school meal standards.

Districts are required to furnish their WP upon request. Enough people asking about this will let the district know that wellness is important to the parents and guardians. It is also possible that a districts WP is out of date or that they do not even have one. Public scrutiny can accomplish a great deal.

A Wellness Policy *must* include the following:
- Measurable goals for nutrition promotion and education, physical activity, and other school-based activities that promote student wellness
- Nutrition guidelines for all foods and beverages sold or made available on school campus during the school day
- Policies for food and beverage marketing
- Requirements that stakeholders be provided opportunities to participate in the development, implementation, and periodic review and update of the wellness policy
- A plan for measuring effectiveness that is measured triennially and made available to the public
- Annual notification informing and updating the public (parents, students, and others in the community) about the content and implementation of the WP
- Designation of one or more district officials or school officials by position or title, to ensure that each school complies with the WP

For any program to be effective and consistent, participating schools must also be supplied with the resources needed to successfully implement it. That being said, Wellness Policies can provide an avenue toward more comprehensive Health Education.[23]

"Whole School, Whole Community, Whole Child (WSCC)" Health Education Model

We do not have to "reinvent the wheel." One model of an integrated school health system is the Centers for Disease Control (CDC) Whole School, Whole Community, Whole Child (WSCC) model. The WSCC framework is student-centered and emphasizes the role of the community in supporting the school, the connections between health and academic achievement, and the importance of evidence-based school policies and practices.

The WSCC model has 10 components:

1. Physical education and physical activity
2. Nutrition environment and services
3. Health education
4. Social and emotional school climate
5. Physical environment
6. Health services
7. Counseling, psychological, and social services
8. Employee wellness
9. Community involvement
10. Family engagement

With careful planning, implementation, and evaluation efforts, use of the WSCC model has the potential to focus family, community, and school education/health resources on increasing the likelihood of better health and academic success for students and improving school and community life in the present and into the future.

WSCC states that structured health education consists of any combination of planned learning experiences that provide the opportunity to acquire the information and skills students need to make quality health decisions. When led by qualified, trained teachers, health education helps students achieve health literacy, adopt health-enhancing behaviors, and promote the health of others via open communication.

Comprehensive school health education for students from pre-K through grade 12 should address a variety of topics such as alcohol and other drug use/abuse, healthy eating and nutrition, mental and emotional health, personal health and wellness, physical activity, safety and injury prevention, sexual health, tobacco use, and violence prevention.

Health education should address the National Health Education Standards (NHES) and incorporate the proven characteristics of an effective health education curriculum.

WSCC identifies that the school nutrition environment provides opportunities to learn about and practice healthy eating through its food and beverage choices, nutrition education, and messages about food within the cafeteria and throughout the school campus.[24,25]

As you can see, there are already methods and pathways available to create opportunities for students to learn about nutrition. We just have to stand up and insist that wellness programs become a priority.

Sending the Message Home

For long-term success, nutrition education programs should involve parents and be implemented in a wide range of settings that include the school and the home. Parent nutrition education can teach healthy lifestyle behaviors and encourage the whole family to make small changes together. Research has proven that this is effective.[26]

The Cafeteria: *Being Consistent*

A comprehensive and consistent nutrition education program should include both the classroom *and* the school cafeteria.

Providing access to healthy foods plays an important role in the academic achievement of students. Students spend much of their time at school and may eat as many as two out of three meals there a day.

Studies show children who eat school meals have better behavior, attendance, and academic performance. These study results were amplified when the students ate both breakfast and lunch at school.[27] Still, many schools do not have a breakfast program, and some administrators want to cut the lunch program altogether.

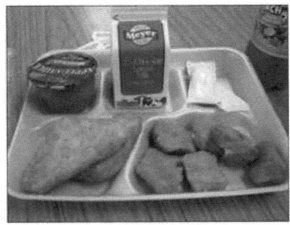

A Standard U.S. School Lunch

In my Nutrition lessons, students often ask, "If this food isn't healthy, then why does the school serve it?" Good question.

Many of these students also say they would eat salad from a fresh, quality salad bar if it were available. Unfortunately, it usually isn't. I have seen poor-quality salads in more than one school cafeteria that don't appeal to the kids. Wilted lettuce, anyone? Again, we are lucky to have *any* school lunch, but really? We *can* do better.

Many schools in California are stepping up to the challenge and are finding that providing healthy and sustainable food can pay off.

Zenobia Barlow, Executive Director of the Center for Ecoliteracy, has seen the power of focusing efforts on healthier school food. Barlow has worked with the Oakland Unified School District, among others, to implement "California Thursdays," a partnership between the Center for Ecoliteracy and participating schools to serve freshly prepared meals using ingredients sourced in California. The program has spread to 71 districts that serve a third of the state's school meals and has inspired similar programs in Minnesota and New York.

California Thursdays include recipes, training, and promotion of unique and tasty menu options. Some popular meals have been halal chili lime chicken and penne pasta with chorizo and kale.[2]

At a middle school in Berkeley, they only serve freshly prepared, locally grown, organic food. They offer lots of fruits and vegetables and healthy versions of pizza and macaroni and cheese using ingredients such as low fat cheeses and local organic milk. The kids love the food and learn that healthy food can taste good.[17]

According to the executive chef for Berkeley Unified, in order to have a healthy meals program, it "takes a community that demands real food that is healthy, nutritious and sustainable in their communities — and they have to stand up for it and make a lot of noise about it."[17]

Arguments against healthier cafeteria food are often cost related. However, studies show that improving the nutritional value of school food doesn't cost anything. One 14-year study showed that, even though the nutritional requirements for school food went up throughout the duration of the study, costs did not.[28]

The results in Berkeley, and other schools like it, are healthier kids who don't get sick as often, have better behavior, and perform better in class.[19]

"Locals Only"

Some schools are "going local" in order to provide fresher, healthier choices to their students. This option also saves money and helps the environment by lessening the length of transport for foods included in the schools' nutrition programs.

Some smaller districts are working collectively to buy local produce. U.C Santa Cruz has worked with 10 school districts in Santa Cruz and Monterey counties to buy local produce through joint contracting.[2]

The Center for Good Food Purchasing in Berkeley encourages large institutions to use their bargaining power to purchase locally produced food as a way to support local workers and local economies. LA Unified has redirected about $12 million into local produce purchases.[2]

Jenn Gerard, former Nutrition Service Director for Monterey Peninsula Unified School District, wanted to increase local access to sustainable food. Gerard reached out to members of the local fishing community and found a willing partner in Real Good Fish CEO Alan Lovewell. Together they created Bay2Tray, which delivers locally caught, fresh, wild fish to local schools as part of California Thursdays. The fish, which is said to be delicious, would have otherwise been discarded as it is often unintentionally caught when fishing for market-friendly black cod. This successful program has expanded to other districts in the area.[2]

The common denominators in each of these programs are the desire and the will to provide healthy food and nutrition education to students. From little to no added cost, we can serve healthier food in schools and positively impact children's health and education.

By providing healthy food in cafeterias, administrators also set the right example as to what the children should be eating — and students are more likely to apply that knowledge to their lives outside of the school setting.

Best Practices

Improving our schools can include learning from those who do it right. Andreas Schleicher, author of *World Class: How to Build a 21st Century School System,* has studied education systems around the world and created the PISA test which measures problem solving, intelligence, and creativity in children. This test helps compare education systems across the world to find what works.[29]

Schleicher advises that, for our education problem to be solved, we need to place more value on education and our children than on consuming (i.e., spending on "stuff" for instant gratification).

Schleicher adds, "Your school system today is your economy tomorrow." Agreed, and that must include nutrition and health education.

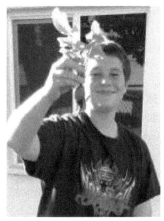

Harvesting Radishes from Our School Garden

Conclusion

Our diabetes and obesity epidemics are a national emergency that must be addressed. We already know solutions such as education and nutrition education work and that effective models exist. So why haven't we applied them? Because an effective strategy prepared to overcome the opposition which is often short sighted and for-profit, has not been designed or implemented on a wide enough scale yet. To succeed, *that* must change.

Human beings are an innovative and determined bunch so we *can* reach our goals, we just need a plan. Solving problems at their root, through comprehensive and inclusive education, is a great plan.

"Give a man a fish and he eats for a day. Teach him to fish and he eats for a lifetime."

We must *learn* how to fish and navigate some rough and greedy waters to achieve sustainable good health for all.

Chapter Eleven

Government: Who's in Charge?

"Bad men need nothing more to compass their ends, than that good men should look on and do nothing."
– John Stuart Mill

For better or worse, the U.S. government has a direct effect on our nutrition and health. Specifically, the EPA, FDA, and USDA all play a role in how food is grown and produced and ensuring food is safe.

Unfortunately, these taxpayer-funded entities, whose job it is to protect the consumer, are falling short in many areas. Though they do good work and are often good-intentioned, they are also being influenced by those with a vested interest in the decisions they make. And that is a *problem*.

In fact, money is deeply affecting government via lobbyists, campaign contributions and political fundraising, and that is one of the biggest barriers to logical solutions, like quality nutrition programs in the U.S.

Money = Power

Politicians receive a lot of money from powerful corporations. To put this in perspective, consider the two top lobbying industries, which spend quite a bit of money trying to "buy" favorable legislation from politicians:

2017 Spending:

1. Pharmaceutical Products: $280,000,000
2. Insurance: $160,000,000[1]

So what about the American people? Who is really protecting and representing us? Who is at the helm of this ship? Actually, *we* are—or at least we should be—but we've been asleep at the wheel.

The government and corporations are accountable to voters, taxpayers, and consumers. Unfortunately, the U.S. government is succumbing to the demands of industry and unnecessarily exposing Americans to unhealthy food and environment.

One way to solve problems is by electing quality leaders. Sadly, too many elected decision makers are there for power and prestige, not the health and welfare of the people. In addition to the constant arguing, blaming, and theatrics in politics today, there is a lack of cooperation, communication, and compromise necessary to find and implement practical solutions for the common good.

Government should look less like a World Wrestling Entertainment ring match and more like reasonable people discussing, debating, compromising, choosing, and implementing workable solutions. We all want to solve our many problems, and there are existing models for how to fix them. Since they work for us, let's "hire" more leaders whose primary goal is problem solving, not benefitting themselves or the interests of a few.

Responsible leaders will be more likely to implement cost-effective solutions such as research for nutritional remedies and education because these programs prevent and solve problems.

The current U.S. political climate is one of "perpetual campaign," in which politicians need to continually please their financial supporters. This leads to a reluctance to make tough, long-term decisions that could negatively impact their benefactors or upset their base. Measures must be taken for politicians to be more responsive to the majority of voters.[2]

Votes equal power, and voters should harness and *use* that power.

The Environmental Protection Agency (EPA)

The purpose of the Environmental Protection Agency (EPA) is to protect the public from environmental health hazards. The EPA is riddled with controversy. There is evidence that the EPA and other governmental agencies are unable and unwilling to hold corporations to account, and that they have even co-conspired to *cover up* potentially damaging information. There are, of course, agency employees trying to do their jobs, but they are often being overridden, their scientific opinions ignored, and research buried, if they conflict with corporate agendas.[3,4,5]

Monsanto Company, also discussed in the Processed Food chapter, is a large and powerful American agrochemical and agricultural biotechnology corporation. Monsanto is the world's largest conventional and GMO seed producer, and manufactures pesticides and the widely-used herbicide "RoundUp." Monsanto is a good example of how industry can influence governmental policies.

Monsanto spends a lot of time and money making sure governmental agencies and legislators approve and support their products. Despite the fact that research shows pesticides and herbicides can cause health problems, and the effects of GMOs in the environment and on human health are largely unknown, Monsanto and the EPA continue to defend these controversial products' and claim they are safe.

Pesticide and herbicide producers are not required to make the full list of their products ingredients public. This makes it difficult for scientists to study the physiological effects of these compounds.[6]

Monsanto spent millions of dollars to defeat a GMO labeling law that would have required GMO foods to be labeled as such so as to inform consumers when they are buying GMO foods.[7] Monsanto won that battle, as the law did not pass.

When I saw this measure on the ballot I found the wording so misleading that, even as a supporter of GMO labeling, I was confused as to which way to vote. Corporations can be extremely tricky, and voters are often confused. Sadly, this is by design.

In early 2017, unsealed court documents revealed there was possible collusion between Monsanto and the EPA to cover up the carcinogenic risks of glyphosate, the main ingredient in Monsanto's RoundUp.[8]

The saga continues as the EPA is now considering the approval of a genetically engineered seed designed to survive glyphosate *and* a highly toxic, older weed killer "2, 4-D," which has been linked to hypothyroidism, suppressed immune function, Parkinson's disease, and cancer, among other ills.[9]

Dissenters

The World Health Organization (WHO) declared Monsanto's glyphosate "probably carcinogenic to humans" in March 2015.[10] There seems to be more clarity on these issues outside of the U.S., probably because there is less pressure and influence by lobbyists on official "opinions."

A California jury ordered Monsanto to pay a record $2 billion in damages to a couple that was diagnosed with non-Hodgkin's lymphoma (NHL) after using RoundUp for years. This verdict was the third time in less than a year that Monsanto was found liable for cancer.

"It's time for the EPA to stand up to Monsanto-Bayer and protect farmers, farm workers, lawn care workers, and consumers," said Alexis Baden-Mayer, political director of the Organic Consumers Association.[4]

There are currently several other cases pending against Monsanto. In fact, more than 13,000 plaintiffs have filed suit against them, alleging they developed non-Hodgkin's lymphoma due to glyphosate exposure.

Monsanto has been losing recent cases, which is a shift from their history of victories. Some cases may even end up in the Supreme Court. At which time, the presidentially appointed judges' beliefs about corporate rights over citizens' rights will matter.

Monsanto was recently acquired by the Bayer Company, and the company name is said to be changing as well. Some think that is to alleviate the negative connotation now associated with the name Monsanto.

he Environmental Working Group (EWG), a consumer watchdog group ited earlier, is also fighting back against Monsanto and other orporations that put profits before public health. This is great news; iowever, these efforts are usually not without retaliation. A Monsanto executive recently attacked EWG, calling their popular "Shopper's Guide o Pesticides in Produce," which warns consumers about Monsanto's products, propaganda.[8]

n summary, the EPA and other governmental entities are not doing their obs and are in need of oversight and intervention, and the public is in need of support from its elected representatives.

The Food and Drug Administration (FDA)

The FDA, along with the USDA, is one of the first lines of defense in protecting the U.S. food supply. However, I think it is safe to say that the defenses are not holding.

The FDA is responsible for ensuring drugs, medical products, food products, and other consumer goods are safe for the American public. The FDA regulates more than $1 trillion in products — almost 10 percent of the country's Gross Domestic Product. But the FDA is said to be underfunded and is therefore vulnerable to influence by wealthy corporations.[11]

In 2009, FDA scientists stated that management is "corrupted and distorted" and that large corporations "ordered, intimidated, and coerced FDA experts to modify scientific evaluations, conclusions, and recommendations in violation of the laws, rules, and regulations, and to accept clinical and technical data that is not scientifically valid."[11]

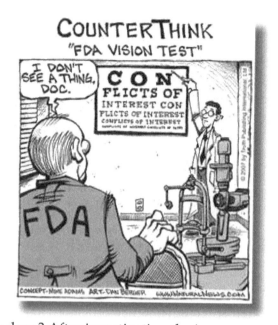

So what can be done? After investigating the issues, some have suggested solutions. For example, the American Academy of Pediatrics (AAP) cites specific actions that could be taken by the FDA and others to provide better oversight of what is allowed to go into our food. AAP's official Policy Statement explains, "The FDA can and should make improvements within the scope of current agency authority, and that ultimately, congressional action may be required" to reform the regulatory process.[12] Of course, this presumes our elected congress people are willing to get things done.

The United States Department of Agriculture (USDA)

The USDA manages various programs related to food, agriculture, natural resources, rural development, and nutrition. The USDA is often conflicted between the goals of the organization – supporting the farming, and agriculture industries and protecting the American public. Often, the industries are supported at the cost of the American Public's health.

The Federal Food Guide

The widely used, federally developed U.S. Dietary Guidelines are issued by the USDA; and Health and Human Services (HHS), which oversees the implementation of numerous health and welfare-related programs, including Medicare and Medicaid.

These dietary guidelines are based, in part, on the advice of an advisory committee made up of experts in the fields of health and nutrition: many of whom have industry conflicts of interest.

On the 2000 Committee, for example, members had past or present ties to two meat associations; four dairy associations and five dairy companies; one egg association; one sugar association; one grain association; five other food companies; six other industry-sponsored associations; two pharmaceutical associations; and 28 pharmaceutical companies.[13]

The committee has been made up of individuals funded by McDonald's, Coca-Cola, the Sugar Association, the American Meat Institute, candy bar companies, and the egg and dairy boards.[13]

The committee bases its recommendations on thousands of pages of published research and public comment, some of which is submitted by the potentially affected industries. Industry efforts *have* made an impact on past and current recommendations. For example, industry influences have resulted in recommendations of consuming more dairy, meat, and grains than many nutrition experts think is optimal, as was discussed in the Healthy Eating chapter.

"There's a great deal of money at stake in what these guidelines say," said Dr. Marion Nestle, one of the experts who helped establish the dietary guidelines.[14]

The evolving USDA Food Guide has issues which have improved over time, and many experts agree that is has helped improve the health of many Americans. However, it is still a multi-faceted concept being influenced by those with their own agendas, therefore like other influential matters, it should be looked at with a scrutinizing eye.

Government-Supported Farms

The U.S. government subsidizes or "helps finance" certain crops to protect against food shortages and ensure farms are successful. The most subsidized agricultural products in the U.S. are corn, soy, wheat, rice, dairy, and livestock. Though initially well intentioned, this has encouraged the overconsumption of certain foods.[15]

Government-supported farms have caused excesses in certain crops and oversaturation of the food market with those ingredients as well as the manipulation of the free market.

For instance, High Fructose Corn Syrup (HFCS) was discovered during a time of an overabundance of corn crops, or more supply than demand.

Despite this engineering accomplishment of sugar's almost-identical twin, after it went to market, they found that consumers still preferred sugar. So, the corn industry pushed (via lobbyists) for sugar tariffs on sugar imports to make HFCS cheaper to purchase. It worked because, soon after, both Coke and Pepsi announced they would convert their products from sugar to high fructose corn syrup. HFCS has since flooded the market.[16] So, once again, pressure and manipulation worked and intervened in the natural supply and demand process.

Corn is also being used for animal feed. Even though the digestive systems of cows are not meant to process corn, that is what they are being fed because there is so much corn available due to these government incentives. If growers listened to the market more and were not just taking directives from the government, the food supply would be more diverse, more natural, and more cows would be raised on pastures eating grass as their bodies were made to do because that is what most consumers want.

There are also "government-supported" soy, wheat, dairy and animal products flooding the market which are manipulated with hormones, pesticides, GMO's, etc., and we are also overconsuming those.

Another downside to the mass production of specific types of food is the practice of "mono-cropping," which is farming the same crop over and over again, resulting in nutrient-depleted soil and food.

Perhaps it is time to revisit the original idea of "food security" and adapt this to meet the goal of "health security."

Big Industry Influences Government

Arizona and Michigan have bowed to the pressure of big industry, and California recently followed suit. California was the latest to try and pass a tax on sugary beverages. Some of these funds could have been directed toward preventing and treating illnesses caused by overconsuming these products. However, the government was essentially blackmailed into dropping the proposed legislation after industry representatives threatened to introduce a statewide bill that would make the passing of *any* new taxes more difficult by raising the voting threshold for *all* local tax measures.[17]

Fearing the ability to fund the government, the state government caved and took the legislation off the table. The industry claims they are only trying to keep the price of groceries down. How thoughtful of them!

After industry lobbyists attended a dinner at the governor's mansion, then-governor Jerry Brown and the California State Legislature approved a ban on any new local soda taxes for 12 years. That is a big win for "Big Beverage."

Tax disincentive programs have been shown to work. A new U.C. Berkeley study found that Berkeley residents decreased their consumption of sugar-sweetened beverages by over 50 percent, while at the same time increasing their water intake by about 30 percent. The effects seem to be cumulative as the numbers increase over time, indicating that people lose their taste for these sugary drinks altogether.[17]

The cities of Berkeley and San Francisco already have soda taxes. San Francisco legislator, Scott Wiener, said, "This industry is aiming a nuclear weapon at government in California and saying, 'If you don't do what we want, we are going to pull the trigger and you are not going to be able to fund basic government services.'"[18]

Americans spend more money on soft drinks than any other food item, which explains the industry's motivation to defend their lucrative products.[19]

Over-consumption of sugary beverages leads to obesity and an increased risk for type two diabetes, heart disease, kidney diseases, non-alcoholic liver disease, tooth decay, and gout, among other health issues.

There is justifiable concern about mass public consumption of sugary beverages, and *something* must be done. So, a food or drink tax is better than nothing.

Though the beverage industry won that very large battle, the war in California continues. State lawmakers are currently pushing a package of bills which include warning labels, size limits, restrictions on where the drinks can be displayed and promoted, and a statewide soda tax to combat the industry efforts.[17] So, stay tuned.

Solutions

There are plenty of cases of private industry interests influencing governmental actions and the U.S. is not the only country dealing with the problems of greed and corruption impacting public health.

The authors of a comprehensive study done on the role of government in nutrition across the globe stated, "Local and national governments have important roles in bringing healthier food and food security to their populations. To our knowledge no country has implemented a full range of updated, comprehensive, and evidence-informed strategies to encourage a healthier and more equitable food system. Given the remarkable health and economic burden of diet-related illness... a coordinated national food and nutrition policy strategy should be a priority for all governments."[20]

To get that done, let's elect people who will respond to the health needs of the American public!

Conclusion

The function of government is to represent public interests. However, those with a vested interest continue to work hard to affect the outcomes of governmental decisions. We are currently being "outgunned" by "big guns" that fight for profits and against public health. However, if enough voters and consumers participate in the processes, they will be "outmanned," "outgunned," and overpowered by our votes and combined dollars.

A balance must be created between individuals, industry, and government. People must push sufficiently on behalf of their own interests—just as corporations and politicians are pushing for theirs.

As John Stuart Mill suggested, it is time for *"good men"* (read: people) to do something.

Chapter Twelve

Societal Solutions:
People Power!

*"If we could give every individual the right amount of nourishment…we would have
the safest way to health."*
– Hippocrates

Many people in this country eat poorly, feel sick, and believe drugs or
"quick-fix" diets can solve their problems. However, the masses are only
responding to what they are told over and over again. We are constantly
bombarded with advertisements for fast food, "junk" food, diet food, and
drugs for everything a poor diet causes. And we have been buying it.

Fast food restaurants spent almost $5 billion on advertising in 2012. To
promote its products, McDonald's alone spent almost triple the
advertising amount as all the fruit, vegetable, bottled water, and
milk advertising budgets combined.[1]

Children see an average of 10,000 "junk" food commercials a year.[2] If
parents spent every meal with their child, that time would only amount
to one-tenth the amount of time children spend viewing television
commercials. To make matters worse, fast-food companies pay famous
athletes, actors, and models to act as their spokespeople. Parents offering
their healthy food have to compete with glamorous, profit-seeking
celebrities pushing not-so-healthy food.

Strapped for Time

Many people today are extremely busy, and there are fast and easy drive-
through restaurants offering plenty of fatty, salty, and sugary comfort
food inside on practically every corner. The average American spends
$1,200 per year on fast food, and 34 percent of children ages 2 to 19
consume fast food on a daily basis.[3]

Strapped for Cash

Many people are struggling financially and think fast-food and other processed "cheap" foods are the best options.

In impoverished areas, unhealthy food is often all that is readily available and seemingly affordable (sometimes real and sometimes perceived affordability). As a result, there are a disproportionate number of poor people who are sick due to diet-related illnesses.

However, the cost of healthy food is often thought to be much higher than it actually is. A study done by Harvard University found that the healthiest diet cost $1.50 more per day than the least healthy one.[4]

The cost of unhealthy food is much greater when you consider the costs of a heart attack, trips to the doctor, copays, medications, and other problems that come from regularly eating unhealthy food.

While studying nutrition in school, I managed to eat healthy on an *extremely* limited budget. It was challenging, but possible because I knew how important it was and had enough know-how to make it happen.

An unhealthy diet negatively impacts learning and education, and education levels usually determine financial stability and success. In short, an unhealthy diet helps perpetuate a cycle of poverty.[5,6]

A Snowball of Sickness

How do you feel after eating a healthy meal? Energetic, clear-minded, focused? Ready to take on the world? How would you feel after a day of chips and soda? This is the difference between healthy and unhealthy food.

Processed, salty, fatty, sugary, chemical-laden foods lack the nutrients the body needs and cause short energy bursts followed by crashes. During an energetic "low," one might be tempted to grab a specially formulated "energy" drink or sugary candy bar for a quick pick-me-up, but these "fixes" only add to the negative cycle, further the chemical imbalances, and make us sick.

Basically, all the flaming hot chips, french fries, and sugary drinks have caught up with us, the go-to solutions of drugs and diets are not working, and our bodies are crumbling under the pressure.

We don't need another fad diet, "new and improved" energy drink, or medication. What we need is to fix the original problem—a poor diet.

What Are Our Priorities?

Every year in the U.S., a lot of money is funneled into "junk" and diet foods, prescription drugs, healthcare (or, more properly named, "sick care") and societal safety nets like welfare, prison, and war.

- Diets: $60 billion[7]
- Drugs: $450 billion[8]
- Fast food: $200 billion[9]
  - Burger King: $10 billion
  - Chick-fil-A: $8 billion
  - Dunkin' Donuts: $8 billion
  - Kentucky Fried Chicken: $4.5 billion
  - McDonalds: $36 billion
  - Pizza Hut: $6 billion[10]
- Healthcare: $3 trillion[11]
- Military spending: $600 billion[12]
- Prison: $200 billion[13]
- Welfare: $500 billion[14]

That is over five *trillion* dollars spent on creating problems and then reacting to them. We can do better.

The U.S. spends $600 billion a year on the military, on war, and on preparing for war, when arguably the most devastating war—in the number of lives lost—is on our health.

The arguments made against preventative programs like nutrition education are often cost related. We have the funds as evidenced by the preceding list. They just need to be invested more wisely.

Reinvesting some of that money into preventive solutions will create another snowball effect—but, in this case, a positive one. More prevention will lead to better health, improvements in learning, and a more prepared and productive populace better able to succeed and contribute to the system via spending in the marketplace and taxes. This is in stark contrast to less healthy, less prepared people who are more reliant on taxpayer-supported safety nets. It simply makes sense, on both a large and small scale, to be proactive.

Solving Whole Problems

Treating issues in a narrow-minded way—such as prescribing a pill without looking at other related factors like nutrition—fails to address the whole problem.

To effectively solve a problem, it is necessary to look at it holistically or as a "whole." For instance, nutrition is inter-dependent on many factors.

Overall human health consists of physical (including nutrition), social, and mental health. These are all related.

When someone's physical health suffers, their mental and social health are also affected. In the High School Health Class I teach, this is taught as three sides of a triangle because each side affects the other. For optimal health, all three aspects of health must be supported and *balanced*.

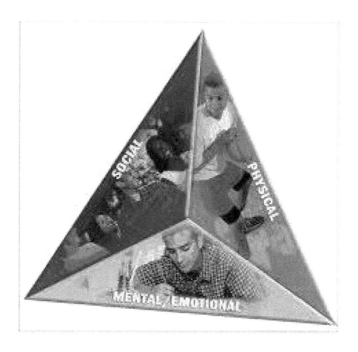

So although nutrition is a part of physical health, it also impacts the other aspects of health. Therefore, I often recommend social and mental health supports to my clients to help them achieve their nutrition goals.

People often have emotional reasons behind their eating habits. For example, when I am working with clients to create an eating plan, personal issues usually come up. Many have feelings, thoughts, and behaviors about food that are tied to emotions and experiences. I have had clients, for example, with alcoholic parents and, though they themselves did not drink, they experienced powerful cravings for certain foods—especially simple carbohydrates.

Many people I have worked with received unhealthy messages from caregivers about body image and how to eat which led to disordered and unhealthy eating.

For effective nutrition counseling and education, everything that affects nutritional health must be considered. To solve any problem, we must onsider "the big picture."

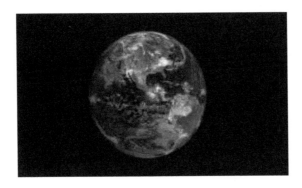

The Planet

Nutrition and the earth are inextricably linked.

The Land

California produces two-thirds of the country's fruits and nuts and more than a third of the vegetables. All across California, where much U.S. food is grown, new homes and everything that goes with them such as shopping centers, auto malls, restaurants, and parking lots, are rising like an ocean swell.

The air, soil, and water quality in these food growing areas are also being affected.

If these careless land grabs continue, the U.S. may become dependent on other countries to supply its produce since much of this urban sprawl is happening on American farmland.

Everyone must do their part to solve our massive societal problems, and as they say, "To whom much is given much is expected." So to repair the imbalances they are creating, perhaps these booming California (mainly high-tech) companies could spread into other states, especially to those that need the jobs and revenue.

Aside from mass housing development, water shortages, record-breaking temperatures, and fires, California also faces serious threats from the effects of a volatile environment.

Data shows that California's farmers are struggling against the impact of climate change including early-blooming crops, heat waves, years of drought, and record-breaking temperatures. Even more severe impacts are predicted, including farmland that is no longer suitable for crops.[15]

The Soil

The goals of modern-day farming practices are to produce food and animals faster, bigger, and more efficiently in order to maximize output and therefore revenue. This has many detrimental effects on soil—the important medium food is grown in.

Soil is made up of air, water, decayed plant residue, organic matter, sand, silt, clay, and minerals. About 24 billion tons of topsoil is lost every year due to agriculture and erosion. To contextualize this, it takes 2,000 years to make 10 centimeters of fertile soil from bedrock naturally.[16]

"Ever since humans developed agriculture, we've been transforming the planet and throwing the soil's nutrient cycle out of balance," said Ronald Amundson, U.C. Berkeley professor of Environmental Science, Policy and Management. "Because the changes happen slowly, often taking two to three generations to be noticed, people are not cognizant of the geological transformation taking place."

Nutrients lost can be captured, recycled, and put back into the ground. Amundson notes, "We have the skillset to recycle a lot of nutrients, but the ultimate deciders are the people who create policy. It's not a scientific problem. It's a societal problem."[17]

Franklin D. Roosevelt said, "The nation that destroys its soil destroys itself."[16]

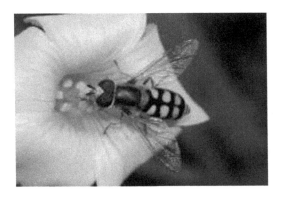

The Bees

Bees transfer pollen and seeds from one flower to another, fertilizing plants so they can grow and produce food. Without bees, many food crops would die off.[18]

Bee populations are declining rapidly, and several types of bees are now on the endangered species list. Some bee species have declined as much as 90 percent over the past two decades.

Threats bees face include pesticides, loss of habitat, diseases and parasites, and climate change.[19] Bees need access to plenty of wildflowers and trees that are free from pesticides in order to thrive and continue to provide sustenance to humans and all the other earthly creatures they support.[20]

The bee problem is another example of humankind's often harsh, invasive, and careless ways which impact our health.

The earth is a healing force in all that it provides: air, water, sustenance, and peace of mind. Remember your last walk in the woods and how it made you feel? We should treat the earth more like an important partner in a relationship to which we are connected, dependent on, and that we *respect.*

Fast vs. Slow Food

The U.S. food supply is unhealthy for many reasons including toxins, nutrient-depleted soil, mono-cropping, and GMOs. Now there is mas development of farmland into housing, shopping malls, and many othe money-making ventures.

Instead of growing food bigger, faster, and primarily for profit, we shoulc return to a slower, more maintainable way of life where peopli participate in smaller, self-sustaining, manageable, holistic, and healthie ecosystems. This would be much healthier for humans, the food we eat and the planet.

Political Solutions

Solving all the problems we face may seem overwhelming, but there are solutions.

We all know there is a major political divide in the U.S. and world. Sadly, some benefit from this division and therefore *want and encourage* it. When people spend time and energy arguing, they're distracted from finding and solving the real problems.

At social gatherings we often hear, "No talking politics. Someone is going to get upset." However, if we don't communicate, how will we solve our problems? We need to *talk* to each other in *healthy* ways. Unhealthy and a general lack of communication are at the root of many of our problems.

Voting can be *a thing*. As it is now, many people don't vote or vote using limited information. Many votes are based on paid advertisements, which are often confusing and misleading. One would not determine the healthiness of a soda, or other profitable product or venture, based solely on the opinion of those who would benefit from its sale. Yet, considering biased information is largely how we determine our laws and political leaders.

There are things that can be done to make the voting process easier. Voters can look to impartial groups and websites dedicated to informing the public about candidates and legislation that can save time and effort.

here are a lot of ways to encourage more people to vote — and that ould be a priority. Voting should be accessible and convenient. Many eople have suggestions for this. Suggestions include making Election ay a National Holiday, expand early voting, allow weekend voting, vote bars and restaurants; and create voter IDs via driver's license or ID pplications.

Personal Solutions

Ve must continue to vote with our voices, dollars, and ballots. Support entle and proactive measures like nutrition education, healthy nadulterated food, green living, and natural healing.

he time is ripe to do something. The public is waking up. If the nomentum continues, we can repair what is broken. Bottom-up forces — he people — can solve the top-down problems if we unite and fight for olutions.

'ersonal and political choices we make every day can reshape the culture nto a healthier one. *We* are the solution.

Obstacles

There will be obstacles.

'or one, there are people who try to discredit alternative methods for nealing our society's poor health. The fact is that many corporations will ose money — and may even go out of business — if the public gets healthy. As a result, corporations are creating campaigns *against* nutrition.

Freedom of speech is an important right; but, if someone is paid to have an opinion to support an agenda, that is "propaganda." Although legal, these misinformation campaigns are hurting people's health.

I have experienced much resistance along my path of working to heal others through education and nutrition — two basic human needs and rights. However, I am still here, still fighting, still standing, and perhaps will tell those stories in another book. I hope you will keep fighting to *and* recruit others!

Whatever the obstacle, it must be overcome if we are to reach our goals of nutritional prosperity and good health.

Conclusion

If someone came to this planet from another, better-run planet, the would probably ask, "Who is in charge here?" What would our answe be?

Our problems will not fix themselves. Earthlings will remain stuck i these cycles of perpetual failure if we continue with the current strategy – or lack thereof. Our strategy should be to find the roots of problems shine light on them, and apply the best remedies to heal them. This wil lead to a change in course from reaction and *failure* to prevention and *success*. The results will be a healthier human race *and* world.

Continue to speak up, stand up, stay informed, and advocate for "the wil of the people." Proponents of practical solutions can win the arguments i they stand up and advocate *persistently*.

If enough people set their minds to it and remain undeterred, we wil *evolve*. Now, I am off to eat my once-in-a-while treat of a doughnut.

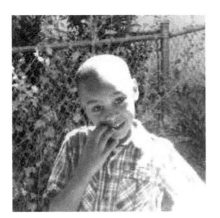

The Indescribable Light of Experiencing
Nutrition Education in the Outdoor Classroom for the First Time
Oakland, CA

Acknowledgments

Thank you to all who contributed to my healing, education, evolving path and this book. Especially Sonia Gaemi and Anna Thomsen for healing me; Muriel Anderson, Ross Edwards, and Amy Roby for editing; Scott Helmer for cover artwork; Jon Erlandson for your tireless support and all of your contributions to this work and my career; Kimberly Ohara-Borowski and Laurie Powell for your selfless contributions to this work and for your incredible work to educate others; my friends and family who continually support me; and to those who blaze a trail, seek answers and never give up; bless you and be *well*.

Appendix A

Healthy Eating Ideas

Here are some of my favorite plant-based meal ideas.

Breakfast: the most important meal of the day!

- Coconut, cashew, or other plant-based yogurt; if unsweetened, sweeten with local honey or maple syrup; add fruit, flax or chia seeds and/or any other creative mix-ins
- Homemade trail mix: I like raw or roasted almonds with dried cranberries
- Oatmeal with nuts, chia, or other seeds; fruit; honey or maple syrup; plant milk; again, get creative!
- Whole-grain bread (e.g., Udi's gluten free, millet, and multi-grain) toasted with almond butter or plant-based buttery spread and fruit spread
- "Grab and go" bars (I prefer Kind brand or other healthy, ethically made bars). Stash them all over so to not be tempted to get a less healthy "fix" at the drive-through!
- Tofu scramble with chopped veggies (garlic, onions, spinach, tomato, avocado, mushrooms, etc.). Add turmeric for yellow color.
- Shredded potatoes (a la hash browns) or chopped potatoes sautéed in vegetable broth. Add chopped garlic, onions, bell peppers, and fresh herbs.
- Plant-based, organic pancakes or french toast (lots of plant-based and vegan recipes are available online). Add bananas or blueberries to batter. Top with maple syrup.
- Plant-based sausage or bacon
- Bagels with plant-based cream cheese, sprinkled with poppy, flax, and/or sesame seeds
- Smoothie made with greens, carrots, ginger, fruit; blend with water, plant milk, or juice

- Cooked brown rice, millet, and/or quinoa topped with shredded apple, cinnamon and plant milk[1]

Lunch

- Mixed green salad with sliced avocado, tomato, onion, cucumber, kidney beans, Italian dressing
- Spinach salad with apple, sunflower seeds, cranberry, balsamic vinaigrette (add marinated sautéed tofu for another source of protein)
- Pasta (I like quinoa, brown rice and others — aside from the overconsumed wheat — to mix it up) with vegan pesto or marinara sauce and mixed vegetables (bell peppers, mushrooms, onions, etc.)
- Tuna salad sandwich (add chopped celery, onions, pickles, vegetable-based mayonnaise) topped with tomatoes and lettuce (serve open face; toast bread and top with lettuce to help keep it together while eating)
- Mixed fruit salad
- Organic, vegan, or vegetarian pizza, loaded with veggies
- All kinds of soups!
- All kinds of salads!
- All kinds of veggies!
- All kinds of herbs!
- All kinds of organic, whole grains (in balance with the other food groups)!
- All kinds of beans, nuts, and seeds!
- All kinds of whole fruit (in balance with other groups, due to sugar content)!

Dinner

- Roasted eggplant, brushed with olive oil and fresh herbs
- Sautéed green beans with Bragg's liquid Amino Acids (tastes like soy sauce)
- Vegan lasagna (my personal favorite vegan food; many recipes can be found online)
- Brown rice or quinoa cooked with vegetable broth

- Bread dipped in olive oil, balsamic vinegar, and herbs
- Baked chopped red or sweet potato, tossed in olive oil and garlic, salt and pepper (tastes like french fries!)
- Roasted asparagus with lemon pepper
- Rice and bean enchiladas (leave out the cheese and meat) add chopped tomato and avocado and a great sauce, accompany with a cold side salad dressed in balsamic vinaigrette; yum!

Snacks

- Cashew, coconut or other plant-based yogurt with blueberries, sweetened with organic honey or maple syrup if unsweetened
- Celery with nut butter
- Carrots with hummus
- Crackers with plant-based cheese

Beverages

- Beth's Spritzer, herbal tea (cold or hot), water with lemon

Dessert

- Fruit
- Sorbet
- Frozen yogurt made with coconut milk
- Plant-based cookies
- Herbal tea with honey (a great way to end the day in a healthy, soothing way!)

Brands

- Amy's, Cedarlane, Gardein and No Evil Foods (wide variety of plant-based meats), Field Roast (plant-based meats and cheeses), Milton's gluten free crackers, Newman's Own, Tofutti (dairy-type products such as cream cheese made with tofu), Udi's, Van's
- Kite Hill for plant-based "cream cheese," Miyoko's, Chao, and Follow Your Heart for a wide variety of plant-based "cheeses"
- Impossible Burger and Beyond Burger for traditional burger appearance and flavor, without the cholesterol

Grocery Stores

- Health Food Stores (have not found one yet that I did not like, though they can be pricey)
- Trader Joe's
- Look for organic, plant-based foods and other "health foods" at many grocery stores and discount stores like Grocery Outlet
- Whole Foods

Certifications

- Fair Trade
- Non-GMO
- Organic
- Vegan

Online Resources

- There are countless recipes online for plant-based versions of just about anything anyone might ever want to make

I support people, companies, places, and products made with care, love, and good ethics. I mainly try to eat organic, minimally processed, or "unadulterated" plant-based food, but there are always exceptions as discussed in my 80/20 plan!

See more healthy meal ideas and share yours at @bethkahn on Twitter, A Nutrition Revolution on Facebook, or on ANutritionRevolution.com.

Good luck! Enjoy a healthy and evolving adventure!

Appendix B

Yearlong Health Class Outline

Introduction to Health — 3 weeks
Defining Health, Health Risk Factors, Taking Responsibility for Your
Health, Decision-Making, Goal Setting, Health Skills

Mental and Emotional Health — 5 weeks
Personality, Emotions, Self-Esteem, Body Image (1-2 days), Eating
Disorders (1-2 days), Stress, Mental Disorders, Suicide

Social Health — 4 weeks
Healthy Family, Peer and Dating Relationships, Communication,
Prejudice, Bullying/Violence/Abuse, Conflict Resolution

Physical Health — 5 weeks
Chronic Diseases, Body Systems, Exercise, Nutrition (2 weeks), Sleep,
Personal Care

Drugs — 5 weeks
Tobacco, Medicines, Alcohol, Illegal Drugs, Preventing Drug
Abuse/Addiction, Refusal Skills

Sexual and Reproductive Health — 7 weeks
Puberty, Sex, Gender, and Sexual Orientation, Anatomy & Physiology,
Abstinence & Healthy Teen Behavior, Pregnancy, Birth Control, Sexually
Transmitted Diseases

Environmental Health and Safety — 5 weeks
Pollution and Global Environmental Issues, Recycling
Infectious Disease, Healthcare System, Safety, Injury Prevention,
Earthquake Preparedness, First Aid, CPR[1]

Appendix C

Student Advocacy

Voices of those who benefit from preventative programs (e.g., students, their families, and guardians) can be effective at advocating for these programs.

During the Community Health section of the yearlong Health Class I teach, my students wrote letters to decision-makers stating whether or not they think a comprehensive Health Class is important and why.

Of the hundreds I collected, the overwhelming majority believed Health class, especially a yearlong comprehensive Health Class, should be taught.

Some of the students' favorite topics included guest speakers who were survivors of abuse, substance abuse, and mental illness; lessons on abstinence, birth control, and healthy relationships; and, of course, nutrition. There were many mentions of planting seeds in our school garden, which the students and I built during my first year teaching high school.

As discussed in the Education chapter, sadly, in February, 2019, the Salinas district school board voted to cut their wonderful, comprehensive, yearlong Health program in half. The change is planned to take effect in August 2020. Most students disagree and are protesting the board's decision.

To learn more about the student-led "Save Health Class" movement, please visit http://bit.ly/savehealthsuhsd.

Here are some examples of student sentiments about the benefits of Health Class. Some of these were sent to the board, and although they made an impact, it wasn't enough. Unfortunately, they did not know they should also be sending them to the Superintendent, who was also apparently pushing for the cut.

Health should be a required high school course so that students get informed about all these things that can help them a lot in their life. It has helped me to not do drugs and to stay abstinent. I have learned multiple ways to say no to drugs. I learned about transmitted diseases, bullying, gender/sexual orientation, eating healthy. Health should be a yearlong course because the more time we have, the more informed we get. I go to high school in Salinas, California. I am currently a sophomore and I say health class is very, very important.

My favorite topic was substance abuse because we had a CHP officer come and talk to us. I think Health should be required because it teaches you things other people won't. I think it should be yearlong because it can't all be packed into just one semester. Health class has helped me by helping me make smart and healthy choices.

I'd like to talk about health class and why it should be a yearlong course and be a required high school course. First of all, you learn a lot of life skills and important things like about growing up, knowing about yourself, avoiding peer pressure, avoid contracting any STDs and avoid making poor decisions.

Kids in high school should get the course, as early as possible which would be freshman year and throughout their high school years they'll have the knowledge about things and apply their knowledge to certain situations. Health has helped me, like think about things I would do, and it's helped me make good decisions.

California high school students should receive a comprehensive health education because not everything that can help us is learned through science classes.

Students need to learn about certain things they can't learn on their own or at home. Some parents are reluctant to have the sex talk. So far I have learned tools that help me avoid peer pressure and I've learned many things about why it is perfectly fine to choose abstinence.

I am from a little known town in California. I am here to talk about the importance of health and how much it can drastically change the community. The mandatory health class at my school has taught me a lot of important facts about my health that I most likely would never have learned elsewhere. Health class should be a countrywide requirement if not at least a CSU requirement.

Health teaches individuals the importance of their bodies, it teaches us how to stay healthy, to help the environment, and so much more. It helps us understand concepts that are important to us, the community, and the planet.

I've learned how to stay healthy, how to help others, how to keep the planet clean and much more. I have no clue why health isn't required as again it provides a lot of information that would be difficult to find otherwise.

Hopefully in the future something changes but as of right now, most of us including myself are not happy with the current policy regarding health class.

Health should be a high school course because teens are at risk if they don't learn about things at home. It should also be a yearlong course so the instructor can go into depth about each topic. Health has helped me because I am sexually prepared if the situation arises and I also know how to care for my health and my community. I enjoyed the presentation rom Planned Parenthood. This has been my favorite presentation because I was able to expand my knowledge of sexual protection. I strongly believe that school boards should make health a requirement.

Thank you for your time.

I think that health class should be required. Health is informational and fun, my favorite activity was the drunk goggles, good thing I did that because it's a big headache. Also, health is so calm it's stress-free, when I learn I don't get knowledge crammed in my head, its super chill, and fun.

Finally, it gives a lot of information like you can say no and you have a voice, and it's important because some people think their alone when they're not they can always call someone, and how to deal with your emotions. It's just better to make the right choices because there are consequences. I just think it would be better to have health all year there is a lot of helpful information.

I believe that health class should be a high school requirement, due to the fact that a majority of high school students are uneducated about health topics. I have learned numerous informative subjects that have prepared me for a healthy future. I advocate for health class being a CSU requirement.

I am a freshman at a Salinas high school. I would like to talk to you about my health class and how it should be a yearlong class. In this past year, I have learned a lot and have had some difficulties.

Although, those difficulties have come to an end; thanks to Ms. Kahn and the health department with all of the hard work they put in to make health class fun, but at the same time informational and healthy.

Honestly, I would consider this a class where you learn about life, self-control, learning about yourself, and learning what happens to your body as you grow.

Also, we learn about avoiding peer pressure, avoiding contracting any STD's, and avoiding making very poor decisions. As students in high school, we should have these types of classes so we can have an idea of what adult life would be like.

It will not be as exact of how adult life is, but just to have an ideal image of what it would be like. For example, peer pressure and self-control. People and parents do say at times "Just say no!" Although, it's not so easy to say "No!" at first because you have the temptation of doing it.

In health class, we go through this topic and the teachers actually explain why this is going on and why we have these kinds of temptations. This topic also comes down to self-control. It really just comes down to self-control because all of the decisions you make has to do with what you think, how you think, and especially the kind of people you hang out with.

How do I comprehend this kind of information already? Because Ms. Kahn and the health department have made plans to try and explain this kind of information. Also, as students in High School, I believe we should have this class as a year-long course because it doesn't only help us, as students, but it also helps our families and friends to understand and learn about yourself and others.

To come into conclusion, health class has helped me a lot, and others, to actually find who we really are. It has helped us to know when it's "too far." And most certainly, it has helped us to be good minded and make good and healthy choices. So says Keri Russell, "Sometimes it's the smallest decisions that can change your life forever."

Thank you and have a wonderful day, Policy Maker.

I am currently taking a yearlong health class. This class is very important for teenagers to help them with what they're going through. A lot of peer pressure goes on during adolescence and because of this class, we've learned ways to say no to drugs, alcohol, and sex. This yearlong course has taught me to take more care of my body and think about the consequences of a situation before doing anything. If the class was shortened, we won't learn all the valuable information to help us throughout our life. It should be a required high school course and remain a year-long course because of the many life skills that we learned and can use for certain situations. It helps make our relationships with family and friends stronger by thinking about others and resolving conflicts in a healthy manner.

Consider the abundant value of this class and the effect it has had on us. Keep health class a yearlong course. Thank you for your time.

I would like to address the topic of making Health a yearlong class and how it should stay yearlong. Health has been a fun class for me, and I believe the rest of the students will agree with that too. My parents don't have the time to sit me down, and teach me how to put a condom on or talk about different types of drugs, and their effect on the human body. On the other hand health has taught me all this valuable information that I believe most people would have a hard time acquiring.

Most students in high-school are going through a lot of stress and depression. When students come to Health class it has made them not as shaky and more open. We learned many ways to relieve stress like going to our school garden once in a while and breathing exercises that help calm our anxiety that we have built up inside. Health being yearlong helped us learned new things that people can't just sit down and talk about at home. All students acquired information that can help others and inspire others to make a good community.

Hello there, I am 14 years old. I'm writing this letter to you to help health classes not become a semester class. My favorite activities in health class are going to the crops to help nature and feel better and meditate. Something you wouldn't get in other classes that can help with stress. My favorite topics are Personality, Emotions, Self-Esteem, Body Image, Eating Disorders, Stress, Mental Disorders, Suicide, Chronic Diseases, Body Systems, Exercise, Nutrition, Sleep, and Personal Care. So it can help freshman learn about sex ed. and help them later in the future. It should be a yearlong course so the health class would not be rushed and for everyone to enjoy health and learn. It helps because it makes families come more together and get along better. I learned about meditation, lots of health issues and how to cure them. Thank you for reading my letter.

Dear Policy Maker,

I am a freshman attending high school, in Salinas, California. In this country with amazing health services, very few places have a proper health education class, let alone the year-long health class I am lucky to be able to attend. I am asking you to keep this year-long class.

This health class is planned to be cut in half, to a single semester. This is a very bad idea for many reasons. The first and biggest one is that the curriculum will be crammed in in only four months, constantly jumping from thing to thing. The second semester adds useful time, that allows for topics to be further explored via methods other than the textbook questions and assessments. This includes guest speakers, videos, Google Slides presentations, exciting exploratory activities (such as visiting the garden, drunk goggles, 'jelly beans' experiments, et cetera) that strengthen one's understanding of the topic at hand, and creates important experiences that, through association, can help one to remember class material in the future.

The advantages of this class are too many for it to become a shell of its current self, and I, as well as the many others teaching and attending this class, will be very disappointed if you cut health class in half.

Appendix D

Community Action Plan

Instead of trying to initiate change at the national or state level, it can be simpler to start at the local level. Here is a plan designed by a health advocate and personal friend (and a really smart guy, who, by the way, first suggested I write a book—thanks, Jon!) that has proven successful. This plan is intended to advocate for healthier cafeteria meals at a district school board meeting; but could easily be adapted to address other topics.

School Board Action Plan

- Attend school board meetings. Invite friends and parents to attend as well. Attendees will soon begin to see what is going on and understand the dynamics of the board power structure.
- Just attending the meetings will set off questions: "Who are you?" and "What do you want?"
- Start by asking questions. Speak at the public input section of the meeting. Get them on the record:
  o Ask: "What does the board plan to do to address the cafeteria menu issues?" Know your facts. Perhaps the district is not meeting the standards—or maybe they *are* meeting the standards, but with minimal compliance. Seek advice and guidance from a local nutritionist or dietitian. Many would be glad to assist.
  o Do research first by obtaining a copy of the current cafeteria scheduled menu. Compare the food offerings with what is required by state and national law.
    ▪ National Nutrition Standards—Nutrition Standards in the National School Lunch and School Breakfast Programs[1]

- California Department of Education — Legislation, Regulations & Policies. Current and proposed legislation, regulations, and policies for child nutrition programs administration[2]
- Check your state department of Education for information on your state.
  - Assume good intentions (e.g., instead of accusing the board of neglecting the nutrition of their students, put it in a positive light and show how the menu can be improved).
  - Offer to serve on a committee to explore the possibilities.
  - Encourage others in the community to get involved.
  - Explore what the board can do to initiate nutritional education. Example:
    - In California: "(5CCR § 15531. Eligibility). Each 'child nutrition entity' defined in section 49530.5 of the Education Code may submit a nutrition education application for funding to the California Department of Education."[3]
    - "(5 CCR § 15534) Procedure for Funding. (a) Each application recommended by the California Department of Education may be approved for funding by the State Board of Education on or before June 15. (b) Payment of expenses incurred by a child nutrition entity shall only be based on actual cost in accordance with the approved project budget."
    - Plan ahead for the first meeting:
      - Explore what is possible — do research.
      - Find out what funding is available through your home state and understand how to get it. Then, when (if?) they say the district cannot afford nutrition education, you can point out that the state will pay for it. It becomes an additional source of income for the district.
      - Explore other funding sources, including non-profits. Look at what non-profit organizations offer funding and invite them to bring their programs to your community. Some possibilities include:
        - Grantwatch.com

- o Grant Helpers.com
- o NewmansOwnFoundation.org
- Local corporations and banks will provide funding to legitimate local community-based groups with worthy causes.
- Be aware of the status of funding availability. Just because the law says the state can provide funding, it may not have budgeted for the program for the current or subsequent year.
- Bring and share details of how other school districts successfully provide nutrition education.
- Your best result may be a task force to explore the situation. Get yourself and your friends on the task force. Try to get someone with knowledge of nutrition and nutritional standards on the committee.
- Give yourselves a name, such as, "Citizens for Nutrition in (your town)."
- Get the word out. Notify the local press of your efforts. If they have some advance notification with an explanation of what you want, they could write an article even if they do not attend. Follow up with them soon after the meeting to share what happened.
- Write letters to the local newspaper or media outlet in which you talk about the next board meeting and express your views. This may engender community support and bring additional people to the meeting.
- Use social media to spread the word.

More resources for improving school food:
- HealthySchoolFood.org
- ForwardFood.org

Resources

Chapter 1, My Story
1. 48 Hours. (2001, November). Out of control. [Television series]. San Francisco, California: CBS.

Chapter 2, Conventional Medicine
1. Warfarin. (n.d.). MedicineNet. Retrieved July 20, 2010, from http://www.medicinenet.com/warfarin-oral/page2.htm.
2. Kerr, G., Bloomfield, Y. (n.d.). Modern ailments ancient remedies: A healing manual. Smithmark.
3. (2018, February 21). Marijuana. Medical News Today. Retrieved November 8, 2018, from https://www.medicalnewstoday.com/articles/320984.php.
4. Fortune Global 500 2008. Top industries: most profitable. (2008, July 21). CNNMoney.com. Retrieved November 27, 2010, from http://money.cnn.com/magazines/fortune/global500/2008/performers/industries/profits.
5. (2018, May 7). National trends in prescription drug expenditures and projections for 2018. Retrieved November 8, 2018, from http://www.ajhp.org/content/early/2018/05/07/ajhp180138.
6. (2009, January 11). How to Understand a Trillion-Dollar Deficit. TIME. Retrieved November 8, 2018, from http://content.time.com/time/business/article/0,8599,1870699,00.html.
7. (2018, March 12). The Top 15 Best-Selling Drugs of 2017. The Lists. GEN. Retrieved November 8, 2018, from https://www.genengnews.com/the-lists/the-top-15-best-selling-drugs-of-2017/77901068.
8. (2018, September 10). Are we really what we eat? Nutrition and its role in the onset of rheumatoid arthritis. NCBI. Retrieved November 8, 2018, from https://www.ncbi.nlm.nih.gov/pubmed/30213695.
9. (n.d.). Diet, Nutrition, and Inflammatory Bowel Disease IBD. Retrieved November 8, 2018, from http://www.crohnscolitisfoundation.org/resources/diet-nutrition-ibd-2013.pdf.
10. (2017, October 12). Antibiotics exposure and risk of inflammatory bowel disease: a systematic review. NCBI. Retrieved November 8, 2018, from https://www.ncbi.nlm.nih.gov/pubmed/29022402.
11. (2018, August 22). Health benefits of taking probiotics. Harvard Health. Retrieved November 8, 2018, from https://www.health.harvard.edu/vitamins-and-supplements/health-benefits-of-taking-probiotics.
12. (2012, September). Heart disease and food. Better Health Channel. Retrieved November 8, 2018, from https://www.betterhealth.vic.gov.au/health/conditionsandtreatments/heart-disease-and-food.
13. Kahzan, O. (2014, June 16). U.S. Healthcare: Most expensive and worst

performing. Retrieved September 18, 2018, from
https://www.theatlantic.com/health/archive/2014/06/us-healthcare-most-
expensive-and-worst-performing/372828.

14. Mateljan, G. (2009, June24). Open letter to President Barack Obama. World's
    Healthiest Foods. Retrieved December 12, 2009, from
    http://whfoods.org/genpage.php?tname=george&dbid=249.

15. Neel, J. (2009, June 9). Medical schools and drug firm dollars. NPR: Health and
    Science. Retrieved October 1, 2009, from http://www.
    npr.org/templates/story/story.php?storyId=4696316&sc=emaf.

16. Adams, K.M., Lindell, K.C., Kohlmeier, M., Zeisel, S.H. (2006, April). Status of
    nutrition education in medical schools. American Journal of Clinical Nutrition,
    83(4):941S–944S.

17. Kamen, B. (Actor), Grapek, J.H. (Director). (2004). ADD/ADHD smart solutions:
    Ways to improve your child's behavior. [Video]. (Available from Associated
    Producers, Inc., Bethesda, Maryland).

18. Daniel, E. (2018, January 26). U.S. Pharma lobbying spend surged to 25.4 m in
    2017. Pharmaceutical Technology. Retrieved September 18, 2018, from
    https://www.pharmaceutical-technology.com/news/us-pharma-lobbying-
    spend-surged-25-4m-2017.

19. (n.d.). Salary for Lobbyist. Salary.com. Retrieved February 1, 2019, from
    https://www1.salary.com/Lobbyist-salaries.html.

20. (2017, January 19). Here are the highest paid lobbyists for 2016. Courier-Journal.
    Retrieved March 8, 2019, from https://www.courier-
    journal.com/story/news/politics/ky-general-assembly/2017/01/19/highest-
    paid-lobbyists-2016/96765912.

21. (2013, November). The Role of Direct-to-Consumer Pharmaceutical Advertising
    in Patient Consumerism. Retrieved November 9, 2018, from
    https://journalofethics.ama-assn.org/article/role-direct-consumer-
    pharmaceutical-advertising-patient-consumerism/2013-11.

22. Moynihan, R., Henry, D. (2006, April). The fight against disease mongering:
    Generating knowledge for action. Public Library of Science Medicine, 3(4).

23. Walker, M. (2003). German cancer therapies (pg. 108). New York: Kensington
    Publishing Group.

24. (n.d.). What is Integrative Medicine? Arizona Center for Integrative Medicine.
    Retrieved December 30, 2018, from
    https://integrativemedicine.arizona.edu/about/definition.html.

25. How to get insurance coverage for dietary counseling. (2005). MedicineNet.
    Retrieved December 1, 2009, from
    http://www.medicinenet.com/script/main/art.asp?articlekey=50695&pf=3&
    page=1.

26. (2010, November 22). Wendell Potter: "My Apologies to Michael Moore and the
    Health Insurance Industry." PR Watch. Retrieved November 9, 2018, from
    https://www.prwatch.org/news/2010/11/9642/wendell-potter-my-apologies-
    michael-moore-and-health-insurance-industry.

27. Sahelian, R. (n.d.). Quackwatch review. Retrieved July 20, 2010, from

http://www.raysahelian.com/quackwatch.html.
28. Eisen, S.C. (2005, October 13). Quackwatch founder Stephen Barrett loses major defamation trial in hometown. Foundation for Health Choice. Retrieved December 15, 2009, from http://www.foundationforhealthchoice.com/victory_barett.html.

Chapter 3, Amino Acids
1. Mindell, E. (1999). Vitamin bible for the 21st century. New York: Warner Books.
2. Balch, P.A. (2006). Prescription for nutritional healing (4th ed.). New York: Avery Publishing.
3. Erectile dysfunction: Alternative treatments. (n.d.). Web MD. Retrieved July 20, 2010, from http://www.webmd.com/ erectile-dysfunction/guide/alternative-treatments-ed.
4. Wong, C. (2007, September 21). Natural remedies for erectile dysfunction. About, Alternative Medicine. Retrieved July 20, 2010, from http://altmedicine.about.com/cs/conditionsetoh/a/ erectiledysfunc.htm.
5. Mahan, L.K., Escott-Stump, S. (2004). Krause's food, nutrition & diet therapy (11th ed.). St. Louis, Missouri: Saunders/Elsevier.
6. Grosvenor, M., Smolin, L. (2002). Nutrition, from science to life. Florida: Harcourt, Inc.
7. Self Nutrition Data. (n.d.). Know what you eat. Retrieved April 4, 2011, from http://nutritiondata.self.com.
8. (2012, April 25). Cost of Buying Viagra at CVS, Walgreens, and Walmart Pharmacy. Retrieved November 9, 2018, from https://www.accessrx.com/blog/erectile-dysfunction/viagra/cost-of-buying-viagra-at-cvs-walgreens-and-walmart-pharmacy.
9. (2016, July). Erectile Dysfunction Drugs Market Worth $3.2 Billion By 2022. Retrieved November 9, 2018, from https://www.grandviewresearch.com/press-release/global-erectile-dysfunction-drugs-market.

Chapter 4, Micronutrients
1. National Institutes of Health. (n.d.). Vitamins: Medlineplus. Retrieved July 20, 2010, from www.nlm.nih.gov/medlineplus/ vitamins.html.
2. Grosvenor, M., Smolin, L. (2002). Nutrition, from science to life. Florida: Harcourt, Inc.
3. Balch, J.F., Balch P.A. (1997). Prescription for nutritional healing (2nd ed.). New York: Avery Publishing Group.
4. Balch, P.A. (2006). Prescription for nutritional healing (4th ed.). New York: Avery Publishing.

Chapter 5, Macronutrients
1. Balch, P.A. (2006). Prescription for nutritional healing (4th ed.). New York: Avery Publishing.
2. (2018, May 9). When it comes to protein, how much is too much? Harvard Health. Retrieved March 12, 2019, from https://www.health.harvard.edu/diet-

and-weight-loss/when-it-comes-to-protein-how-much-is-too-much.

3. Grosvenor, M., Smolin, L. (2002). Nutrition, from science to life. Florida: Harcourt, Inc.
4. (2018, August 13). The truth about fats: the good, the bad, and the in–between. Harvard Health. Retrieved March 9, 2019, from https://www.health.harvard.edu/staying-healthy/the-truth-about-fats-bad-and-good.
5. (n.d.). Trans fat: Avoid this cholesterol double whammy. Mayo Clinic. Retrieved November 9, 2018, from https://www.mayoclinic.org/diseases-conditions/high-blood-cholesterol/in-depth/trans-fat/art-20046114.
6. United States Department of Health and Human Services and United States Department of Agriculture. (2010). Dietary guidelines for Americans. Retrieved February 3, 2011 from http://www.cnpp.usda.gov/Publications/DietaryGuidelines/2010/PolicyDoc/PolicyDoc.pdf.
7. (2018, February 22). How Much Cholesterol Should I Have Per Day? Healthline. Retrieved November 9, 2018, from https://www.healthline.com/health/high-cholesterol/rda.
8. Self Nutrition Data. (n.d.). Know what you eat. Retrieved December 27, 2009, from http://www.nutritiondata.com/ foods-0.html.
9. Agnel, P., Sims. E., Houston, J., Konieczny, R. (2017, August 14). 63 Million Americans exposed unsafe drinking water. USA Today. Retrieved September 19, 2018, from https://www.usatoday.com/story/news/2017/08/14/63-million-americans-exposed-unsafe-drinking-water/564278001.
10. (n.d.). The Facts. Plastic Oceans Foundation. Retrieved November 15, 2018, from https://plasticoceans.org/the-facts.
11. (2018, November 2). How Much Water Should I Drink? Healthline. Retrieved November 15, 2018, from https://www.healthline.com/health/how-much-water-should-I-drink.
12. State of the air. (2010). American Lung Association. Retrieved November 20, 2010, from http://www.stateoftheair.org/2010/ key-findings.

Chapter 6, Healthy Eating

1. US News and World Report (November 2017): "The Trouble with Lectins." Stacey Colino. Retrieved July 28, 2018 from https://health.usnews.com/wellness/food/articles/2017-11-29/the-trouble-with-lectins.
2. Powell, L. (2018, November). Email interview.
3. (2015, August 10). Meat and Poultry Labeling Terms. USDA Food Safety and Inspection Service. Retrieved November 29, 2018, from https://www.fsis.usda.gov/wps/portal/fsis/topics/food-safety-education/get-answers/food-safety-fact-sheets/food-labeling/meat-and-poultry-labeling-terms/meat-and-poultry-labeling-terms
4. (n.d.). Pastured Raised Grass Fed Chicken. Circle C Farm. Retrieved November 9, 2018, from https://www.circlecfarmfl.com/collections/pastured-raised-grass-

fed-chicken.

5. (2012, May 1). How Big Are Your Dinner Plates And Why It Matters: Eat Out, Eat Well. Retrieved November 16, 2018, from https://eatouteatwell.com/how-big-are-your-dinner-plates-and-why-it-matters.
6. (2016, April 28). The History of Portion Sizes: How They've Changed Over Time. Your Weight Matters. Retrieved November 9, 2018, from https://www.yourweightmatters.org/portion-sizes-changed-time.
7. (2018, January 3). U.S. News Reveals Best Diets Rankings for 2018. US News and World Reports. Retrieved November 9, 2018, from https://www.usnews.com/info/blogs/press-room/articles/2018-01-03/us-news-reveals-best-diets-rankings-for-2018.
8. (2018, January 3). Keto, Whole30 diets rank last on one best diets of 2018 list. ABC News. Retrieved November 9, 2018, from https://abcnews.go.com/Health/keto-whole30-diets-rank-best-diets-2018-list/story?id=51953127.
9. (2007, February 1). Is Fasting Healthy? WebMD. Retrieved November 9, 2018, from https://www.webmd.com/diet/features/is_fasting_healthy.
10. (n.d.). Nutritional Update for Physicians. Plant-Based Diets. Retrieved November 29, 2018, from http://www.thepermanentejournal.org/issues/2013/spring/5117-nutrition.html.
11. (n.d.). 7 Tips for Clean Eating – Eating Well. Retrieved November 9, 2018, from http://www.eatingwell.com/article/78846/7-tips-for-clean-eating.
12. United States Department of Agriculture. (2009). National nutrient database for standard reference, release 22. Retrieved December 30, 2009, from http://www.nal.United States Department of Agriculture.gov/fnic/foodcomp/search.
13. (n.d.). World Health Organization (WHO). Physical Activity and Adults. Retrieved November 16, 2018, from http://www.who.int/dietphysicalactivity/factsheet_adults/en.

Chapter 7, Processed Food

1. (2019, February 11). Eating ultraprocessed foods increases your risk of ... - New York Post. Retrieved February 26, 2019, from https://nypost.com/2019/02/11/eating-ultraprocessed-foods-increases-your-risk-of-early-death-study.
2. United States Department of Agriculture. (2009). National nutrient database for standard reference, release 22. Retrieved December 30, 2009, from http://www.nal.United States Department of Agriculture.gov/fnic/foodcomp/search.
3. (2018, December 18). Safer Food for a Healthier You. Retrieved November 9, 2018, from https://www.webmd.com/diet/features/safer-food-healthier-you.
4. (2014, November 12). EWG's Dirty Dozen Guide to Food Additives. EWG. Retrieved November 11, 2018, from https://www.ewg.org/research/ewg-s-dirty-dozen-guide-food-additives.

5. (n.d.). Reduce Antibiotic Misuse in Livestock. NRDC. Retrieved November 11, 2018, from https://www.nrdc.org/issues/reduce-antibiotic-misuse-livestock.

6. (2017, November 17). World Health Organization Urges Farmers to Stop Overusing Antibiotics in Livestock. EWG. Retrieved November 11, 2018, from https://www.ewg.org/enviroblog/2017/11/world-health-organization-urges-farmers-stop-overusing-antibiotics-livestock.

7. (2017, October 3). List of Vegetables That Are Genetically Modified. Livestrong.com. Retrieved November 11, 2018, from https://www.livestrong.com/article/428500-list-of-vegetables-that-are-genetically-modified.

8. (2018, April 23). Are G.M.O. Foods Safe? The New York Times. Retrieved November 11, 2018, from https://www.nytimes.com/2018/04/23/well/eat/are-gmo-foods-safe.html.

9. (2019, February 6). High-Fructose Corn Syrup: Just Like Sugar, or Worse? Healthline. Retrieved February 22, 2019, from https://www.healthline.com/nutrition/high-fructose-corn-syrup-vs-sugar.

10. (2015, January 19). Scientists Find High Fructose Corn Syrup Is as Bad For You as You Might Think. Retrieved February 22, 2019, from https://www.ecowatch.com/scientists-find-high-fructose-corn-syrup-is-as-bad-for-you-as-you-migh-1882000552.html.

11. (n.d.). Sneaky Names For MSG (Check Your Labels!). Hungry for Change. Retrieved November 11, 2018, from http://www.hungryforchange.tv/article/sneaky-names-for-msg-check-your-labels.

12. (2017, January 29). Pictures: What You Should Know About Processed Meat. WebMD. Retrieved November 29, 2018, from https://www.webmd.com/food-recipes/ss/slideshow-processed-meats.

13. (n.d.). Food Additives and Child Health. From the American Academy of Pediatrics. Retrieved November 29, 2018, from http://pediatrics.aappublications.org/content/142/2/e20181408.

14. (n.d.). WHO. Q&A on the carcinogenicity of the consumption of red meat and processed meat. Retrieved March 7, 2019, from https://www.who.int/features/qa/cancer-red-meat/en.

15. (n.d.). What is the Difference Between Pesticides, Insecticides and Herbicides? Retrieved May 15, 2019, from http://www.llojibwe.org/drm/greenteam/pesticides_Article.pdf.

16. (2017, March 13). How Much Toxic Roundup Are You Eating? Good Housekeeping. Retrieved November 29, 2018, from https://www.goodhousekeeping.com/health/diet-nutrition/a20706601/how-much-toxic-roundup-are-you-eating.

17. (n.d.). Glyphosate. EPA. Retrieved May 17, 2019, from https://www.epa.gov/ingredients-used-pesticide-products/glyphosate.

18. (2018, June 28). Decades of deceit on glyphosate. Pesticide Action Network. Retrieved November 11, 2018, from http://www.panna.org/blog/decades-deceit-glyphosate.

19. (n.d.). Pesticides. National Institute of Environmental Health Sciences. NIH. Retrieved November 11, 2018, from https://www.niehs.nih.gov/health/topics/agents/pesticides/index.cfm.

20. (2018, March 1). IARC Monograph on glyphosate. Retrieved February 23, 2019, from http://www.iarc.fr/en/media-centre/iarcnews/2016/glyphosate_IARC2016.php.

21. (2018, February 7). How Toxic is the World's Most Popular Herbicide Roundup? The Scientist. Retrieved November 29, 2018, from https://www.the-scientist.com/news-opinion/how-toxic-is-the-worlds-most-popular-herbicide-roundup-30308.

22. (2017, March 1). Trans fat: Avoid this cholesterol double whammy. Mayo Clinic. Retrieved November 11, 2018, from https://www.mayoclinic.org/diseases-conditions/high-blood-cholesterol/in-depth/trans-fat/art-20046114.

Chapter 8, Research

1. (n.d.). Scientific method. Oxford Reference. Retrieved January 28, 2019, from http://www.oxfordreference.com/view/10.1093/oi/authority.20110803100447727.

2. Neel, J. (2009, June 9). Medical schools and drug firm dollars. NPR: Health and Science. Retrieved October 1, 2009, from http://www.npr.org/templates/story/story.php?storyId=4696316&sc=emaf.

3. Perlis, R.H., Perlis, C.S., Wu, Y., Hwang, C., Joseph, M., Nierenberg, A.A. (2005, October). Industry sponsorship and financial conflict of interest in the reporting of clinical trials in psychiatry. American Journal of Psychiatry, 162(10):1957-60.

4. (2017, April 19). Too many studies have hidden conflicts of interest. A new tool makes it easier to see them. Vox. Retrieved November 11, 2018, from https://www.vox.com/2017/4/19/15350048/pubmed-publishing-conflicts-of-interest-funding-information.

5. Folic acid may improve asthma, allergies. (2009, May). The Natural Standard Research Collaboration. Retrieved December 12, 2009, from http://naturalstandard.com.

6. Tabak, C., Wijga, A.H., de Meer, G., Janssen, N.A.H., Brunekreef, B., Smit, H.A. (2005, October 21). Diet and asthma in Dutch school children. Thorax, 20`06, 61(12):1048–1053. Published online, doi: 10.1136/thx.2005.043034. Retrieved December 12, 2009, from http://www.ncbi.nlm.nih.gov/pmc/articles/PMC2117046/?report=abstract.

7. Bateman, B., Warner, J.O., Hutchinson, E., Dean,T., Rowlandson, P., Gant, C., Grundy, J., Fitzgerald, C., Stevenson, J. (2004, June). The effects of a double-blind, placebo controlled, artificial food colourings and benzoate preservative challenge on hyperactivity in a general population sample of preschool children. Arch Dis Child, 89(6):506-11.

8. Carter, C.M., Urbanowicz, M., Hemsley, R., Mantilla, L., Strobel, S., Graham, P.J., Taylor, E. (1993, November). Effects of a few food diet in attention deficit disorder. Arch Dis Child, 69(5):564-8.

9. Doggett, M.A. (2004). ADHD and drug therapy: Is it still a valid treatment?

Journal of Child Health Care, 8(1):69-81.

10. Boris, M., Mandel, F.S. (1994, May). Foods and additives are common causes of the attention deficit hyperactive disorder in children. Ann Allergy, 72(5):462-8.

11. Akhondzadeh, S., Mohammadi, M., Khademi, M. (2004, April 8). Zinc sulfate as an adjunct to methylphenidate for the treatment of attention deficit hyperactivity disorder in children. B.M.C. Psychiatry, 4:9.

12. Otero, G., Pliego-Rivero, F.B., Contreras, J.R., Fernandez, T. (2004, July 25). Iron supplementation brings up a lacking P300 in iron deficient children. Clinical Neuropsychology, 115(10):2259-2266.

13. Young, S.N. (2002, January 22). Clinical nutrition 3: The fuzzy boundary between nutrition and psychopharmacology. CMAJ, 166(2):205–209. Retrieved November 25, 2010, from http://
www.ncbi.nlm.nih.gov/pmc/articles/PMC99276/?tool=pubmed.

14. Vitamin C may affect blood pressure. (2009, January). The Natural Standard Research Collaboration. Retrieved December 12, 2009, from http://naturalstandard.com.

15. Algae for blood clots. (2007, August). The Natural Standard Research Collaboration. Retrieved December 12, 2009, from http://naturalstandard.com.

16. Acupuncture for blood pressure. (2007, August). The Natural Standard Research Collaboration. Retrieved December 12, 2009, from http://naturalstandard.com/news/news200708006.asp.

17. Phytoestrogens for bone health. (2007, August). The Natural Standard Research Collaboration. Retrieved December 12, 2009, from http://naturalstandard.com.

18. University of California at Davis, Nutrition Department. (2006, February). Clinical nutrition course 116b: Nutrition and cancer.

19. Morley, K.L., Ferguson, P.J., Koropatnick, J. (2007, June 18). Tangeretin and nobiletin induce G1 cell cycle arrest but not apoptosis in human breast and colon cancer cells. Cancer Lett, 251(1):168-78.

20. Foltz-Gray, D. (2003, Jan., Feb.). Good Food — The Magic of Mushrooms. Alternative Medicine, pp. 39-45.

21. Chi-Fung Chan, G., Man-Yuen Sze, D. (2009). Supplements for immune enhancement in hematologic malignancies. Hematology, pp. 313-319. Retrieved August 5, 2010, from http://asheducationbook.hematologylibrary.org/cgi/content/ full/2009/1/313.

22. Pomegranate for prostate cancer. (2009, May). The Natural Standard Research Collaboration. Retrieved December 12, 2009, from http://naturalstandard.com.

23. Shanafelt, T.D., Call, T.G., Zent, C.S., et al. (2009, May 26). Phase I trial of daily oral polyphenon E. in patients with asymptomatic rai stage 0 to II chronic lymphocytic leukemia. Journal of Clinical Oncology, 10;27(23):3808-14.

24. (2013, March 18). Is There Any Other Anti-Cancer Botanical Compound As Exciting As Curcumin? Retrieved November 11, 2018, from https://integrativeoncology-essentials.com/2013/03/is-there-any-other-anti-cancer-botanical-compound-as-exciting-as-curcumin.

25. Chen. C., Kao. C., Liu. C. (2018, September 12). The cancer prevention, anti-inflammatory and anti-oxidation of bioactive phytochemicals targeting the TLR4

signaling pathway. Retrieved September 26, 2018 from,
https://www.ncbi.nlm.nih.gov/pubmed/?term=30213077.

26. Llewellyn, D.J., Langa, K.M., Lang, I.A. (2009, September). Serum 25-hydroxyvitamin D concentration and cognitive impairment. U.K. Journal of Geriatric Psychiatry, Neurology, 22(3):188-95.

27. Tveden-Nyborg, P., Johansen, L.K., Raida, Z., et al. (2009, September). Vitamin C deficiency in early postnatal life impairs spatial memory and reduces the number of hippocampal neurons in guinea pigs. American Journal of Clinical Nutrition, 90(3):540-6.

28. Meyers, S. (2000). Use of neurotransmitter precursors for treatment of depression. Alternative Medicine Review, 5(1):64-71.

29. Marx, W., Moseley, G., Berk, M., & Jacka, F. (2017). Nutritional psychiatry: The present state of the evidence. *Proceedings of the Nutrition Society, 76*(4), 427-436. doi: 10.1017/S0029665117002026.

30. Balch, P.A. (2006). Prescription for nutritional healing (4th ed.). New York: Avery Publishing.

31. (2017, December). Addressing the Antinomy Between Health Education and Health Literacy in Advancing Personal Health and Public Health Outcomes. NCBI. Retrieved November 11, 2018, from https://www.ncbi.nlm.nih.gov/pubmed/29096417.

32. How to get insurance coverage for dietary counseling. (2005). MedicineNet. Retrieved December 1, 2009, from http://www.medicinenet.com/script/main/art.asp?articlekey=50695&pf=3& page=1.

33. United States Department of Agriculture, Expanded Food and Nutrition Education Program. (2006). Impact data. Retrieved January 13, 2009, from http://www.nifa.usda.gov/nea/food/ efnep/pdf/2006_impact.pdf.

34. (2014, May). Health and Academic Achievement. CDC. Retrieved November 11, 2018, from https://www.cdc.gov/healthyyouth/health_and_academics/pdf/health-academic-achievement.pdf.

35. Adams, K.M., Lindell, K.C., Kohlmeier, M., Zeisel, S.H. (2006, April). Status of nutrition education in medical schools. American Journal of Clinical Nutrition, 83(4):941S-944S.

36. United States Department of Agriculture, Food and Nutrition Information Center, National Agriculture Library. (2004, March). Nutrition, learning and behavior in children: A resource for professionals. Baltimore, Maryland. Retrieved April 13, 2006, from http://www.nal.UnitedStatesDepartmentofAgriculture.gov/fnic/service/learnpub.html.

37. Severson, K. (2010, September 24). Told to eat its vegetables, America orders fries. NY Times. Retrieved September 27, 2010, from http://www.nytimes.com/2010/09/25/health/policy/25vegetables.html?page wanted=1&_r=2.

38. (2013). The Context for Change: Nutrition Education in the K-12 Curriculum. NCBI; NIH. Retrieved November 11, 2018, from

https://www.ncbi.nlm.nih.gov/books/NBK202126.
39. Nikiphorou, E., Philippou, E. (2018, November). Are we really what we eat? Nutrition and its role in the onset of rheumatoid arthritis. Autoimmunity Reviews, 17(11): 1074-1077. 1568–9972. https://doi.org/10.1016/j.autrev.2018.05.009.
40. Lakhan, S.E., Vieira, K.F. (2008). Nutritional therapies for mental disorders. Nutrition Journal, 7:2 doi: 10.1186/1475-2891-7-2, online at: http://www.nutritionj.com/content/7/1/2.
41. Potential weight-loss effects of African mango. (2009, April). The Natural Standard Research Collaboration. Retrieved December 12, 2009, from http://naturalstandard.com.

Chapter 9, The Brain

1. Lakhan, S.E., Vieira, K.F. (2008). Nutritional therapies for mental disorders. Nutrition Journal, 7:2 doi: 10.1186/1475-2891-7-2, online at: http://www.nutritionj.com/content/7/1/2.
2. Meyers, S.(2000). Use of neurotransmitter precursors for treatment of depression. Alternative Medicine Review, 5(1):64-71.
3. Balch, P.A. (2006). Prescription for nutritional healing (4th ed.). New York: Avery Publishing.
4. (2018, April 22). Mental Illness in Children. Retrieved November 11, 2018, from https://www.webmd.com/anxiety-panic/mental-health-illness-in-children#1.
5. Centers for Disease Control and Prevention. (2010, May 25). Attention deficit hyperactivity disorder: Data and statistics in the United States. Retrieved November 27, 2010, from http://www. cdc.gov/ncbddd/adhd/data.html.
6. Schnoll, R., Burshteyn, D., Cea-Aravena, J. (2004, November 2). Nutrition in the treatment of attention deficit hyperactivity disorder: A neglected but important aspect. Applied Psychophysiology and Biofeedback, 28(1):63-75. 1090-0586 (Print) 1573-3270 (Online).
7. Lawlis, F. (2004). The ADD answer. New York: Penguin Group.
8. Kamen, B. (Actor), Grapek, J.H. (Director). (2004). ADD/ ADHD smart solutions: Ways to improve your child's behavior. [Video]. (Available from Associated Producers, Inc., Bethesda, Maryland).
9. Commercial and pipeline insight: ADHD. (n.d.). Retrieved November 28, 2010, from https://www.leaddiscovery.co.uk/ reports/1055/Commercial_and_Pipeline_Insight_ADHD.
10. ADD and ADHD drug revenues. (n.d.). Retrieved January 13, 2009, from www.leaddiscovery.co.uk.com.
11. DeGrandpre, R. (1999). Ritalin nation. New York: W.W. Norton and Company.
12. Doggett, M.A. (2004). ADHD and drug therapy: Is it still a valid treatment? Journal of Child Health Care, 8(1):69-81.

Chapter 10, Education

1. (2017, May 3). Obesity and Overweight. CDC. Retrieved November 11, 2018,

from https://www.cdc.gov/nchs/fastats/obesity-overweight.htm.
2. (2017, February 9). How California is reinventing school lunch. University of California. Retrieved November 11, 2018, from https://www.universityofcalifornia.edu/news/how-california-reinventing-school-lunch.
3. Wooten, M., Stitizel, K. (2003). Nutrition education, a position statement. The National Alliance for Nutrition and Activity. Washington, D.C.
4. Centers for Disease Control and Prevention. (n.d.). Diabetes and women's health across the life stages: A public health perspective. Retrieved February 3, 2011, from http://www.cdc. gov/diabetes/pubs/women/index.htm.
5. American Association for Health Education. (2008). Health literacy. Retrieved December 9, 2009, from www.aahperd.org/aahe.
6. U.S. Department of Education, National Center for Education Statistics. (2009). The nations report card. Retrieved February 3, 2011, from http://nces.ed.gov/nationsreportcard/pdf/ main2009/2011451.pdf.
7. (2018, October 17). Teachers in America: No matter where they work, they feel disrespect. USA Today. Retrieved November 11, 2018, from https://www.usatoday.com/in-depth/news/nation/2018/10/17/teachers-appreciation-pay-union-jobs-schools-education/1509500002.
8. Study: 7.3 million in U.S. prison system in '07. (2009, March 2). CNN. Retrieved November 26, 2010, from http://edition. cnn.com/2009/CRIME/03/02/record.prison.population/index.html?iref=allsearch.
9. (2013). The Context for Change - Nutrition Education in the K-12 Curriculum. NCBI; NIH. Retrieved November 11, 2018, from https://www.ncbi.nlm.nih.gov/books/NBK202126.
10. U.S. Department of Education, National Center for Education Statistics. (1996). Nutrition education in public elementary and secondary schools. Retrieved April 28, 2011, from http://nces. ed.gov/pubs/web/96852.asp.
11. National Alliance for Nutrition and Activity. (2005, March). Model of local school wellness policies on physical activity and nutrition. Washington, D.C.
12. U.S. Department of Education, National Center for Education Statistics. (2000). Nutrition Education in Public School Elementary School Classrooms, K-5. Retrieved April 28, 2011, from http://nces.ed.gov/pubs2000/2000040.pdf.
13. (n.d.). Life Lab - Santa Cruz. Retrieved February 22, 2019, from https://www.lifelab.org.
14. (n.d.). Center for Ecoliteracy. Retrieved February 22, 2019, from https://www.ecoliteracy.org.
15. Waters, A. (2009, September 21). A forum: Food for all, how to grow democracy. The Nation, pp. 12-13. Online at: http://www. thenation.com/article/healthy-constitution.
16. (n.d.). The Edible Schoolyard Project. Retrieved November 29, 2018, from https://edibleschoolyard.org.
17. Jewsbury, M., Owen, J. (2010, June 27). School gardeners perform better in the

classroom. The Independent. Retrieved October 9, 2010, from http://www.independent.co.uk/life-style/ house-and-home/gardening/school-gardeners-perform-better-in- the-classroom-2011528.html.

18. Ellis, K. and Rosenfeld, L. (Producers, Writers and Directors). (2009, August 26). A healthy school lunch. [Video]. (Available from Edutopia, San Rafael, California). Retrieved July 20, 2010, from www.edutopia.org/school-lunch-nutrition-berkeley-video.

19. Ernst, J. (2010, May 2). Five minutes in the green can boost mood. Reuters. Retrieved August 5, 2010, from http://www.reuters.com/article/idUSTRE6401Y620100502.

20. (2014, May). Health and Academic Achievement. CDC. Retrieved November 11, 2018, from https://www.cdc.gov/healthyyouth/health_and_academics/pdf/health-academic-achievement.pdf.

21. (n.d.). Appropriate Practices in School-Based Health Education. SHAPE America. Retrieved November 11, 2018, from https://www.shapeamerica.org/uploads/pdfs/Appropriate-Practices-in-School-Based-Health-Education.pdf.

22. (n.d.). World Health Organization (WHO). Global school health initiative. Retrieved November 29, 2018, from https://www.who.int/school_youth_health/gshi/en.

23. (n.d.). Local School Wellness Policy. California Department of Education. Retrieved November 11, 2018, from https://www.cde.ca.gov/ls/nu/he/wellness.asp.

24. (2015, August 19). Components of WSCC. CDC. Retrieved November 11, 2018, from https://www.cdc.gov/healthyschools/wscc/components.htm.

25. (2015, August 2). Using the Whole School, Whole Community, Whole Child Model: Implications for Practice. Wiley Online Library. Retrieved November 11, 2018, from https://onlinelibrary.wiley.com/doi/pdf/10.1111/josh.12304.

26. Kelsey, R. "Parent Nutrition Education and the Influence on Family Lifestyle Behavior Changes" (2012). All Graduate Theses and Dissertations. 1216. Retrieved October, 27 2018, from https://digitalcommons.usu.edu/etd/1216.

27. United States Department of Agriculture, Food and Nutrition Information Center, National Agriculture Library. (2004, March). Nutrition, learning and behavior in children: a resource for professionals. Baltimore, Maryland. Retrieved April 13, 2006, from http://www.nal.usda.gov/fnic/service/learning.pdf.

28. United States Department of Agriculture, Food and Nutrition Service. (n.d.). Meal cost study. Retrieved July 19, 2010, from http://www.fns.usda.gov/ora/menu/Published/CNP/FILES/MealCostStudy.pdf.

29. Zakaria, F. (Interviewer). (2018, September 2). Interview of Andreas Schleicher. [Television broadcast interview]. New York, New York: CNN.

Chapter 11, Government

1. (2018, October 24). Lobbying. OpenSecrets. Retrieved November 11, 2018, from https://www.opensecrets.org/lobby.
2. Zakaria, F. (Interviewer). (2018, September 2). Interview of Dr. Dambisa Moyo. [Television broadcast interview]. New York, New York: CNN.
3. (2019, June 13). Trump's EPA Has a Monsanto Problem. In These Times. Retrieved July 9, 2019, from http://inthesetimes.com/article/21904/monsanto-lawsuits-glyphosate-cancer-regulatory-capture.
4. (2019, June 26). EPA Urged to Put Public Health Over Monsanto Profits by Banning Cancer-Linked Glyphosate. Retrieved July 9, 2019, from https://www.commondreams.org/news/2019/06/26/epa-urged-put-public-health-over-monsanto-profits-banning-cancer-linked-glyphosate.
5. (2019, June 23). Agriculture Department buries studies showing dangers of Climate Change. Politico. Retrieved July 9, 2019, from https://www.politico.com/story/2019/06/23/agriculture-department-climate-change-1376413.
6. (2019, February 25). Soda taxes have healthful effects. PressReader. Retrieved February 26, 2019, from https://www.pressreader.com/usa/san-francisco-chronicle/20190225/281672551229507.
7. (2018, June 29). California bows to beverage industry, blocks soda taxes. NBC News. Retrieved November 11, 2018, from https://www.nbcnews.com/health/heart-health/california-bows-beverage-industry-blocks-soda-taxes-n887796.
8. (2018, February 7). How Toxic is the World's Most Popular Herbicide Roundup? The Scientist. Retrieved November 17, 2018, from https://www.the-scientist.com/news-opinion/how-toxic-is-the-worlds-most-popular-herbicide-roundup-30308.
9. (2017, December 14). Americans Spend More on Soft Drinks Than Any Other Food Item. Huffington Post. Retrieved November 11, 2018, from https://www.huffpost.com/entry/sugar-sweetened-beverages-are-the-1-category-of-food_b_5a32a844e4b0b0232b691bf7.
10. (n.d.). FDA and Regulation of GMOs. American Bar Association. Retrieved November 11, 2018, from https://www.americanbar.org/content/newsletter/publications/aba_health_esource_home/aba_health_law_esource_1302_bashshur.html.
11. (2018, October). EWG Glyphosate Survey, Sign For Good: Surveys. Retrieved November 11, 2018, from https://surveys.signforgood.com/glyphsurvey.
12. (2017, March 13). How Much Toxic Roundup Are You Eating? Good Housekeeping. Retrieved November 17, 2018, from https://www.goodhousekeeping.com/health/diet-nutrition/a20706601/how-much-toxic-roundup-are-you-eating.
13. Dietary Guidelines: Advisory Committee Conflicts of Interest. NutritionFacts.org. Retrieved July 11, 2019, from https://nutritionfacts.org/video/dietary-guidelines-advisory-committee-conflicts-of-interest.

14. (2018, March 1). IARC Monograph on glyphosate. Retrieved February 23, 2019, from http://www.iarc.fr/en/media-centre/iarcnews/2016/glyphosate_IARC2016.php.
15. Adams, M. (2009, January 12). FDA is deeply "corrupted and distorted," claim its own scientists in protest letter. Natural News. Retrieved January 13, 2009, from http://www.naturalnews.com/News_000655_FDA_scientists_Obama_corruption.html.
16. (n.d.). Food Additives and Child Health. From the American Academy of Pediatrics. Retrieved November 29, 2018, from http://pediatrics.aappublications.org/content/142/2/e20181408.
17. (2016, January 8). Food Industry Lobbying and U.S. 2015 Dietary Guidelines. Time. Retrieved November 11, 2018, from http://time.com/4130043/lobbying-politics-dietary-guidelines.
18. (2017, November 27). The Government Has Been Meddling in Food and Nutrition for a Long Time. Retrieved February 22, 2019, from https://fee.org/articles/the-government-has-been-meddling-in-food-and-nutrition-for-a-long-time.
19. (2016, July 18). Does Subsidizing Crops We're Told to Eat Less of Fatten Us Up? NPR. Retrieved November 11, 2018, from https://www.npr.org/sections/thesalt/2016/07/18/486051480/we-subsidize-crops-we-should-eat-less-of-does-this-fatten-us-up.
20. (n.d.). Role of government policy in nutrition — barriers to and opportunities for healthier eating. The BMJ. Retrieved February 22, 2019, from https://www.bmj.com/content/361/bmj.k2426.

Chapter 12, Societal Solutions

1. (2013, November 5). Fast Food Facts 2013. Robert Wood Johnson Foundation. Retrieved November 11, 2018, from https://www.rwjf.org/en/library/research/2013/11/fast-food-facts-2013.html.
2. Food fight: childhood obesity and the food industry. (2003, July 17). Nightline. [Television series]. New York, New York: ABC.
3. (2015, September 16). Products, Data Briefs: Number 213. September 2015. CDC. Retrieved November 11, 2018, from https://www.cdc.gov/nchs/products/databriefs/db213.htm.
4. (2013, December 5). Eating healthy vs. unhealthy diet costs about $1.50 more per day. Retrieved November 11, 2018, from https://www.hsph.harvard.edu/news/press-releases/healthy-vs-unhealthy-diet-costs-1-50-more.
5. Chilton, M., Chyatte, M., Breaux, J. (2007, October). The effects of poverty and food insecurity on child development. Indian J Med Res, 126:262-272.
6. Campbell, C. (2001, August 21). Health education behaviors models and theories — a review of the literature part 1. Mississippi State University, Coordinated Access to the Research and Extension System (C.A.R.E.S.). Retrieved October 2009, from http://msucares.com/health/health/appa1.htm.
7. Reisner, R. (n.d.). The diet industry: A big fat lie. Business Week. Retrieved

December 28, 2009, from http://www.businessweek. com/debateroom/archives/2008/03/the_diet_indust.html.

8. (2018, May 7). National trends in prescription drug expenditures and projections for 2018. Retrieved November 11, 2018, from http://www.ajhp.org/content/early/2018/05/07/ajhp180138.

9. Baertlein, L. (2010, November 12). San Francisco mayor to veto curb on fast-food toys. Reuters. Retrieved February 3, 2011, from http://www.reuters.com/article/2010/11/12/us-fastfood-toys-idUSTRE6AB4UG20101112?sp=true.

10. (2017, August 2). Most successful fast food chains in America. Business Insider. Retrieved November 11, 2018, from https://www.businessinsider.com/most-successful-fast-food-chains-in-america-2017-8.

11. Kahzan, O. (2014, June 16). U.S. Healthcare: Most expensive and worst performing. Retrieved September 18, 2018, from https://www.theatlantic.com/health/archive/2014/06/us-healthcare-most-expensive-and-worst-performing/372828.

12. (2017, July 7). What NASA could do with US military's budget. Business Insider. Retrieved November 11, 2018, from https://www.businessinsider.com/what-nasa-do-with-us-military-budget-2017-7.

13. Webb hearing explores cost of incarceration in the United States. (2007, October 4). Retrieved July 20, 2010, from http://webb. senate.gov/newsroom/pressreleases/2007-10-04-03.cfm.

14. Chantrill, C. Welfare Spending. U.S. Government Spending. Retrieved January 6, 2011, from http://www. usgovernmentspending.com/welfare_chart_40.html.

15. The Desert Sun. James, I. February, 2018, "California Agriculture Faces Serious Threats from Climate Change, Study Finds."

16. (2016, December 11). 10 Facts About Healthy Soil. Food Tank. Retrieved November 11, 2018, from https://foodtank.com/news/2016/12/10-facts-healthy-soil.

17. (2015, May 7). Soil depletion threatens global food security. University of California. Retrieved January 8, 2019, from https://www.universityofcalifornia.edu/news/soil-depletion-threatens-global-food-security.

18. (n.d.). Bees. NRDC. Retrieved February 20, 2019, from https://www.nrdc.org/sites/default/files/bees.pdf.

19. (2017, March 22). First U.S. Bumblebee Officially Listed as Endangered - Latest Stories. Retrieved November 11, 2018, from https://news.nationalgeographic.com/2017/03/bumblebees-endangered-extinction-united-states.

20. (2018, January 27). Honeybees Help Farmers, But They Don't Help The Environment. NPR. Retrieved November 11, 2018, from https://www.npr.org/sections/thesalt/2018/01/27/581007165/honeybees-help-farmers-but-they-dont-help-the-environment.

Appendix A
1.   Powell, L. (2018, November). Email interview.

Appendix B
1.   August, 2018. Health Department Pacing Calendar. Salinas Union High School District.

Appendix D
1.   (2012, January 26). Department of Agriculture. Government Publishing Office. Retrieved December 1, 2018, from https://www.gpo.gov/fdsys/pkg/FR-2012-01-26/pdf/2012-1010.pdf.
2.   (n.d.). Legislation, Regulations, & Policies. Nutrition (CA Department of Education). Retrieved December 1, 2018, from https://www.cde.ca.gov/ls/nu/lr.
3.   (n.d.). Article 3. Nutrition Education. California Code of Regulations. Retrieved December 1, 2018, from https://govt.westlaw.com.

About the Author

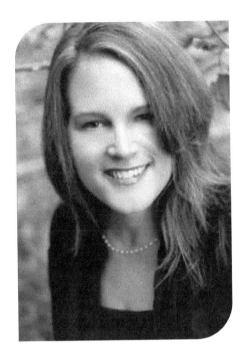

Elizabeth Kahn earned a Bachelor of Science degree in Clinical Nutrition from the University of California at Davis, and a Health Science Teaching Credential from Brandman University. She teaches Culinary, Food Safety, and Health Science in Salinas, California, and maintains a private nutrition consulting practice where she counsels and educates families, businesses, and individuals about nutrition and wellness. For more information visit: www.anutritionrevolution.com.

CPSIA information can be obtained
at www.ICGtesting.com
Printed in the USA
BVHW032247081121
621159BV00013B/107